WARD LOCK

FAMILY HEALTH GUIDE

MENOPAUSE & HRT

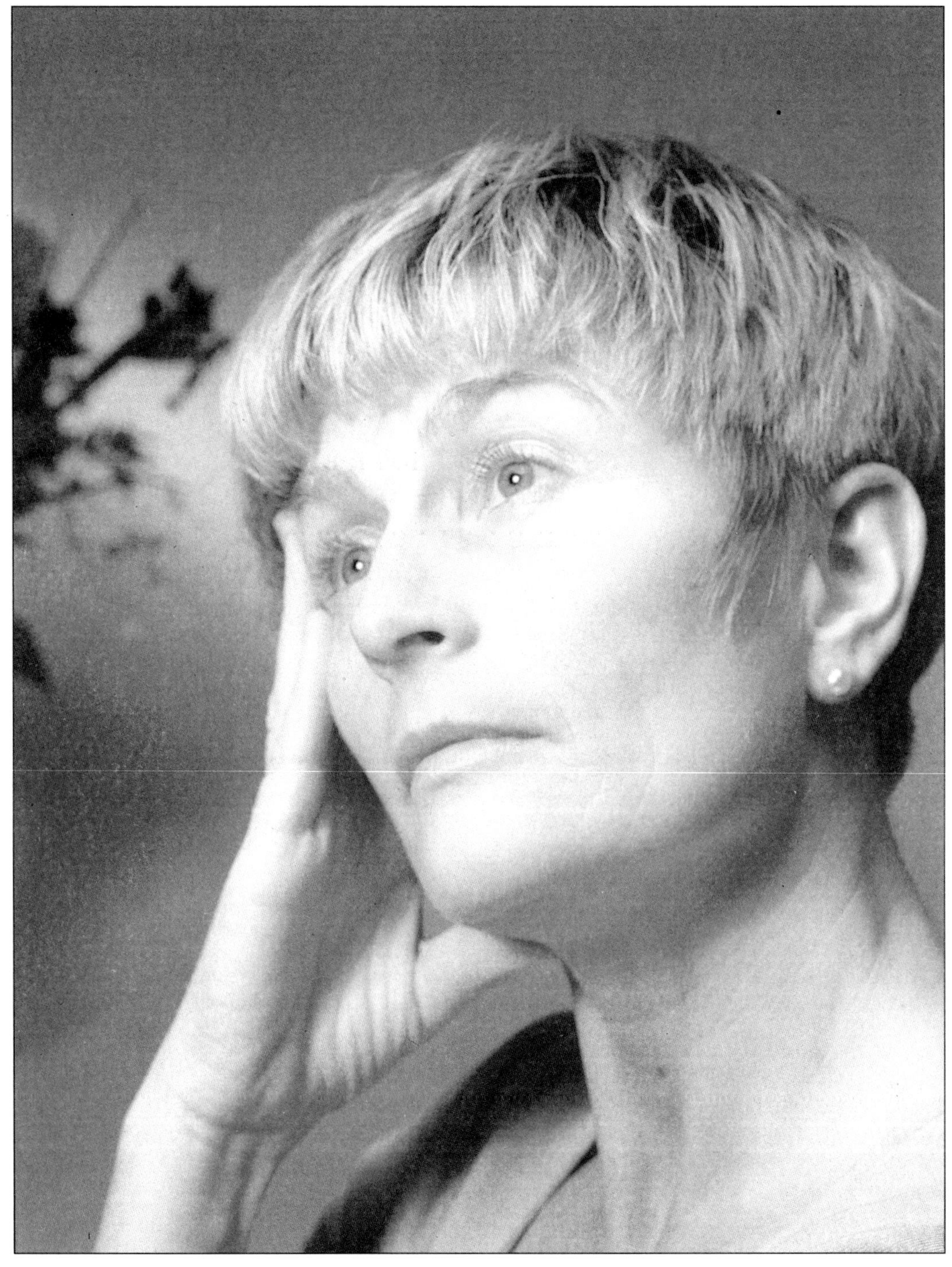

WARD LOCK

FAMILY HEALTH GUIDE

MENOPAUSE & HRT

HEATHER KIRBY

IN ASSOCIATION WITH
THE MARIE STOPES CLINIC

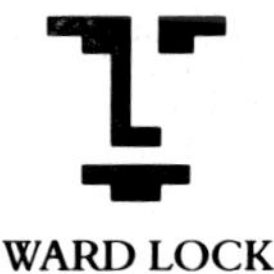

WARD LOCK

Heather Kirby
Heather Kirby is an experienced journalist who writes on a wide range of topics for national newspapers and women's magazines in the UK. She is a regular contributor on health matters for The Times and the Daily Mail, and is the author of a book on healthy eating.

A WARD LOCK BOOK

First published in the UK 1994
by Ward Lock
Villiers House
41/47 Strand
London
WC2N 5JE

A Cassell Imprint

Designed and produced
by SP Creative Design
147 Kings Road, Bury St Edmunds, Suffolk, England

Editor: Heather Thomas
Art director: Rolando Ugolini
Illustrations: Rolando Ugolini

Distributed in the United States
by Sterling Publishing Co., Inc.
387 Park Avenue South, New York, NY 10016-8810

Distributed in Australia
by Capricorn Link(Australia) Pty Ltd
2/13 Carrington Road, Castle Hill, NSW 2154

A British Library Cataloguing in Publication Data block for this book may be obtained from the British Library.

ISBN 0 7063 7255 7

Printed and bound in Spain

Acknowledgements
The publishers would like to thank Dr John Moran and Dr Vanessa Mooney for their help in producing this book, and also the following organisations and individuals for providing photographs:
Cover photograph: The Image Bank (Juan Alvarez)
Fresh Fruit and Vegetable Information Bureau: pages 55, 57, 58, 60
Sandoz Pharmaceuticals: pages 30, 50
Sea Fish Industry Authority: page 65
Mark Shearman: page 32
Wyeth Laboratories: pages 2, 44, 46

Contents

Introduction

Some women don't have one, or, at least, they don't notice it. One day they had periods as usual, and the next – nothing. A few think they have missed a couple of months and assume that the menopause is upon them only to discover that they are, in fact, pregnant. Such is life.

However, for some women the menopause brings with it tremendous problems. These may include heavy and irregular bleeding, painful periods, a dry vagina, night sweats and depression. A generation ago all those things would have been seriously distressing and although they are no less tiresome today, there is plenty that women can now do to help themselves. Suffering in silence is not, thank goodness, something that we do in the 1990s.

The word 'menopause' is derived from two Greek words: 'men' meaning month, and 'pausis' meaning cessation. It is not something that happens overnight. There are three stages that may last as long as ten years, and the general medical term given to the transition from reproductive to post-reproductive age is the climacteric.

1 The peri-menopause signals the declining function of the ovaries. This is when your periods become irregular and other symptoms like hot flushes start to occur.

2 The menopause is when everything that is going to happen is happening.

3 The post menopause is recognised as the time when you have not menstruated for twelve months.

Statistically twenty five per cent of all women pass through the menopause without any problems at all. Another twenty five per cent have serious difficulties and the majority are half-way between. Although there is an inevitable sadness about reaching this threshold, when nature dictates that you cannot have another baby, the gloom passes. And there are, in my opinion, more gains than losses.

Chapter one

Check your biological clock

At birth a baby girl is born with an average of half a million eggs in her ovaries ready to give birth herself when the time comes. Gradually the number diminishes until by puberty she will have approximately 75,000 and by the time she is forty there will be as few as 5,000. Menopause occurs when there are about 1,000 eggs left. Precisely when the ovary is going to have no eggs left and therefore will cease to eject them during menstruation it is impossible to predict. Some ovarian activity continues after menopause.

Some women experience what is called a premature menopause which usually means under the age of 40. Having a hysterectomy generally advances the age at which ovarian failure occurs, so women can experience menopausal symptoms over a decade before the hands of a normal biological clock would strike. Women who have had treatment for radiotherapy and chemotherapy for certain types of leukaemia may have a premature menopause; so can infertile women and women who have had endometriosis.

Women who smoke heavily or who live at high altitudes often begin their menopause early. One theory regarding smokers is that the contents of cigarette smoke causes the liver to destroy oestrogen. The other suggests that nicotine reduces the blood supply to the ovary which, lacking nourishment, may shrivel. Although the age at which girls begin their periods has steadily been getting lower, the average age for women beginning the menopause has remained constant.

For the majority, the time when menopause begins has changed little over the centuries. The big difference between now and earlier ages is that we live a lot longer. Female life expectancy in the western world is now 80 and therefore, on average, a woman can expect to spend 30 years, or 40

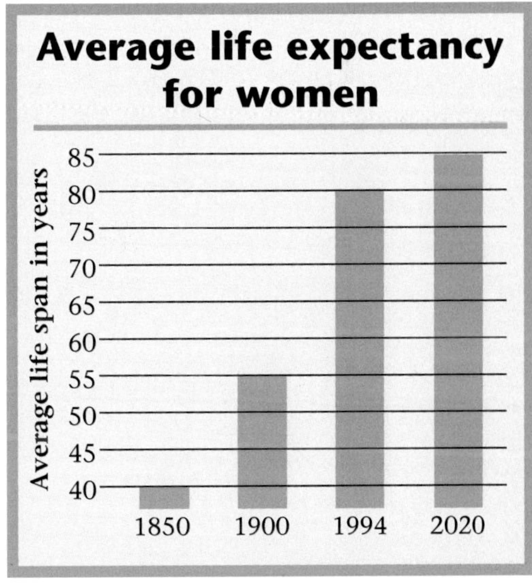

Check your biological clock

When does menopause start?

There is no rite of passage for the menopause. No symbolic key of the door, no date when you can throw a big party to celebrate the occasion. Yet you are about to enter an exciting new era, a time which is full of promise and possibilities. Now you are old enough to know what you don't want, you can think about what you do want. Draw a circle round any of these suggestions which you can feasibly take up to make the most of 'the change':

- Alter my eating habits.
- Learn a language.
- Become a local councillor.
- Take a degree at the Open University.
- Join the Ramblers Association.
- Compete in a gardening competition.
- Join a choir.
- Learn to sail, windsurf, hang-glide.
- Write a book.
- Publish a magazine.
- Change my car.
- Join a health club.
- Buy a bicycle.
- Treat myself to a monthly massage.
- Do voluntary work.
- Learn to play an instrument.
- Consult a doctor.
- Take hormone replacement therapy.

And then set a date when you are going to wind up your psychological clock for a fresh start. Good luck!

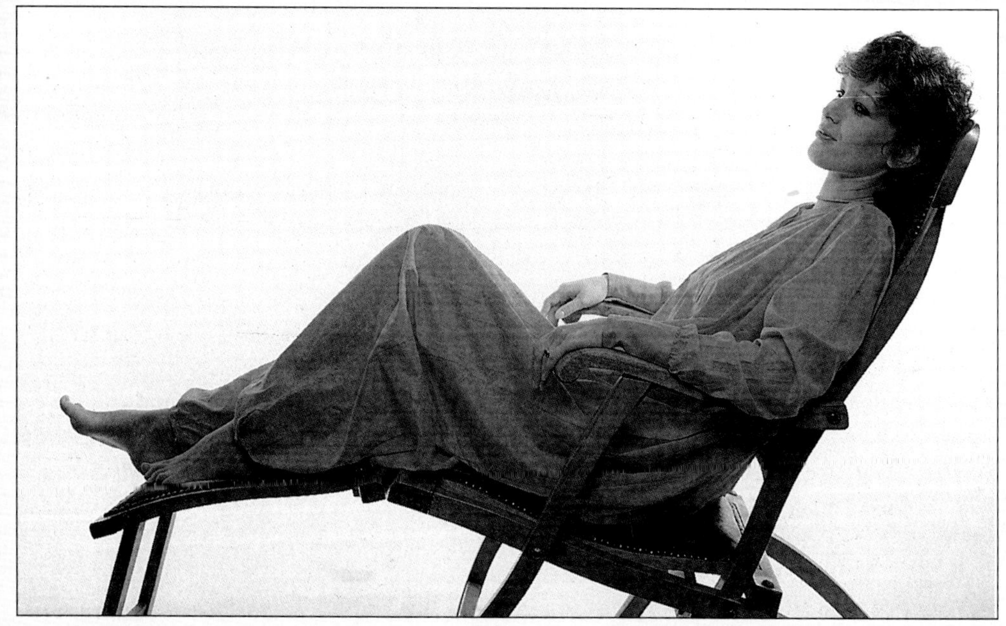

Hormonal changes and menopause symptoms

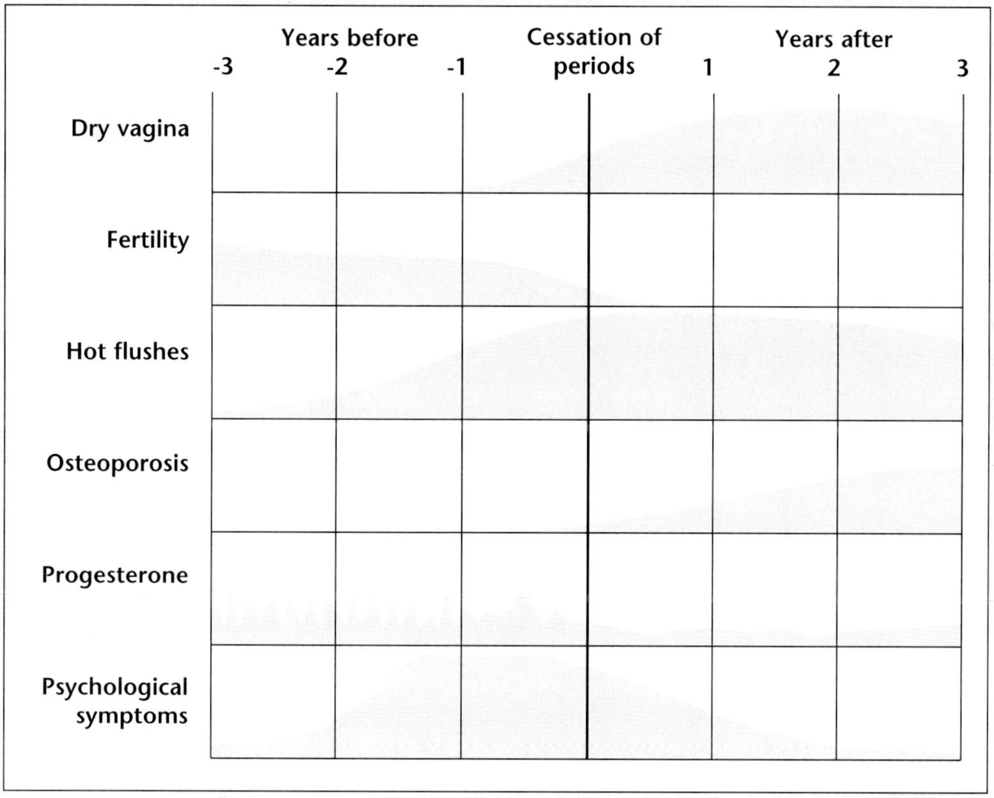

Years before
-3 -2 -1
Cessation of periods
Years after
1 2 3

Dry vagina

Fertility

Hot flushes

Osteoporosis

Progesterone

Psychological symptoms

per cent of her active life, in the postmenopausal stage.

The table below is an indication of just how much things have changed for women.

It is crucial, therefore, that we are able to enjoy those extra years in the best of health. Quality time is what women want. There are almost 10 million of us over the age of 50 in the UK, representing 17 per cent of the population. In the next 20-30 years there will be a 50 per cent increase in the number of women over 85; presumably, since you are reading this book you are around the menopause age so you could well be one of them. To make the most of the rest of your life you need to be as healthy as modern medicine can make you.

Most women suffer from a cluster of complaints so it is worth spending some time working out which ones are making your biological clock tick faster. The acute symptoms, hot flushes, night sweats and insomnia, called vasomotor disturbances, occur first together with many of the psychological problems and it is likely they are, to an extent, interdependent.

A social disease?

We live in a world dominated by flattering images of women. Models parading down the catwalks of the world's fashion capitals with impossibly perfect figures feature constantly in all our daily newspapers. Their hair is glossy, their skin glows, their legs go on forever and their smiles are dazzling.

Advertisements don't sell their products with lines like, "I couldn't care less what brand of floor cleaner I use so long as it does the job well and quickly." They generally show a seriously houseproud woman conducting meaningful conversations – as if the green goo she is sloshing around the kitchen is a matter of great concern to her.

Do you identify with them? The likely answer is No. Because this vision of one half of the world's population is constructed mostly by the other half – men.

For decades now our culture has paid an almost pagan homage to youth and beauty. The inevitable consequence was that the menopause, that period when we commence our 'decline into sexual obsolescence' as a male medic so charmingly put it, became a social disease to be dreaded. The 'menopausal woman' was a term of derision.

Thankfully this attitude is at last changing – not least because women today refuse to be deemed dustbin fodder just because they have reached a certain age. Instead, they are taking the subject by the scruff of its neck and declaring, "You are not getting the better of me!"

And, as you will discover, the menopause doesn't have to be as awful as you have been led to believe – far from it. Just think of all the women who are now well past their menopausal age: Joan Collins, Elizabeth Taylor, the Queen. Have they let the 'change of life' cramp their style? Exactly. Anyway, in the real world women have fat hips and thin hair, friendly wrinkles and flaky skin, sunny dispositions and scruffy ovens. Let's be proud, not apologetic. The well-known anthropologist Margaret Mead coined the phrase 'post-menopausal zest' and I hope in the following pages to describe why and how you should regard the autumn of your days as the liberating phase.

Chapter two

Help, what is happening to me?

Some of the most troublesome symptoms of the menopause are not life threatening but they are extremely embarrassing as well as very painful. If you have not experienced them yourself or through a relative or friend, it is hardly possible to imagine just how debilitating some of them can be.

Unfortunately, many menopausal problems occur at the same time as other worries are crowding in on you: hugely traumatic things like divorce or redundancy or just trying events like moving house or children sitting exams. There is often precious little space left over for you to get the sympathy and support you may need.

However, you are obviously one of those people who believes her fate is in her own hands and does something about it – which is half the battle. And, hopefully, you will discover enough in the following pages to help you overcome whatever it is about the menopause that is worrying you – and that is the other half of the battle won.

Bladder bother

A not uncommon symptom of the menopause, women often discover to their dismay, is an inability to control their water works. An unexpected sneeze or cough, laughing, running or jogging are all normal things you do every day which can suddenly

Quick tips

- Wedge toilet tissue over the urethral opening to absorb drips.
- Go to the toilet more often.
- Train yourself not to sneeze or cough unexpectedly.
- Always carry spare tights/pants.
- Keep a supply of vaginal wipes in your handbag so you minimise the possibility of an infection.
- Lose weight because obesity may exacerbate the problem.
- Stop smoking because inevitably you will cough more often.
- Do pelvic floor exercises.

cause a little urine to escape.

The urethra orifice, which is lined with a similar membrane to the vagina, can become dry and less efficient during the menopause. Cystitis and fungal infections may also occur. The drop in your oestrogen levels can cause a slackening of your pelvic floor muscles and, in consequence, control of the bladder mechanism. The resultant 'accidents' are usually referred to as 'stress incontinence'.

Irregular bleeding

It is important to distinguish between irregular and heavy bleeding. Irregular bleeding means your normal period with the usual amount of blood loss but the cycle may shorten to 21 or 24 days, or you may miss one or even two months. Women vary greatly in the way their menstruation cycles peter out and, so long as you are not experiencing a flood, there is no cause for alarm. Just be careful not to throw contraceptive caution to the winds too soon because that is how many 'accidents' happen.

Heavy bleeding, on the other hand, can be a symptom of something more serious and should be investigated by your doctor. Women may become seriously anaemic and so tired they are unable to carry on their daily activities. A flood can be very embarrassing, especially for women who

Heavy bleeding

Heavy bleeding can be caused by:

- Stress which is something we can rarely avoid these days but it tends to be an isolated incidence of a particularly stressful event which causes heavy bleeding. A long journey can be stressful enough to cause heavy bleeding. If it happens more than once consult your doctor.
- Fibroids are non-malignant tumours which are oestrogen-dependent and usually shrink and often disappear after the menopause. But while such drastic chemical changes are going on they can grow to a troublesome size causing heavy bleeding or abdominal pains. A pelvic ultrasonography can confirm their presence and they can sometimes be removed by a nyomectomy or a total hysterectomy. You can leave them and accept that they are going to increase in size, but they can be monitored and if they cause heavy bleeding you can have them removed.
- Cancer of the endometrium (lining of the womb) would cause unusual breakthrough bleeding and needs immediate medical attention but it can normally be treated successfully, though only by a hysterectomy.

suffer the distress of suddenly "coming on" in the middle of a busy store or station platform. If this should happen to you, there is absolutely nothing you can do other than make your way as calmly as you can to the nearest toilet. And console yourself with the thought that it has happened to many others before you. Once you have survived the experience you will be prepared. I know a woman who never goes anywhere without a complete change of clothing – which she has needed three times so far.

Hot flushes and night sweats

Hot flushes are probably the commonest – and certainly one of the most uncomfortable – symptoms of the menopause. It is estimated between 75-85 per cent of women encounter the phenomenon in some degree. For a few they are so bad they have to sleep in towelling robes or get up and change the sheets. On average they last for two years but occasionally can go on far longer than that. Moderate symptoms would be up to six flushes per day and up to two sweats each night.

What causes them?

- Chemical and hormonal changes in the body.
- Particularly a sudden drop in oestrogen.
- Increased sensitivity to temperature.
- Breakdown in communication between brain and skin.
- Blood vessels near the skin surface dilate and blood pours through the vessels, bringing heat to the skin.
- Oestrogen levels are either too high or too low.

What to do

- Take as many clothes off as you can.
- Treat yourself to a battery-operated fan.
- Pat temples, behind ears and wrists with cold water or eau de cologne.
- Try not to be embarrassed as this will make you blush anyway, though that's easier said than done!.
- Avoid hot caffeine drinks, over-heated rooms, alcohol, nicotine, sugar and emotional upset (again, easier said than done).
- Do not let yourself get underweight because that can affect your oestrogen output.
- Wear cotton next to your skin.
- Learn relaxation exercises.
- Consult your doctor because a hormone replacement could easily eliminate the problem.

Help, what is happening to me?

No longer a woman?

There are some absurd notions voiced about the menopause. Just because your ovaries have stopped functioning doesn't mean you are any less of a woman. Yet we are sometimes treated as if we are past our sell-by date. Middle-aged men are often fussed and fauned over but middle-aged women are sometimes treated as if they are invisible. It is as if, once the child-producing machine has packed in, our usefulness ceases.

Some of the changes to our reproductive organs cause severe distress but the vast majority of women I talk to welcome the menopause. It is one of the compensations of growing older. It means goodbye to periods which, even if they were never painful, were often a nuisance. The knowledge they have to put up with periods once again is one of the main reasons women give for refusing to take hormone replacements. Unless their menopausal symptoms are so bad anything would be better than enduring them, some women say thanks, but no thanks.

If being less of a woman means no more fear of becoming pregnant and getting signals from your body to be on red alert every twenty-eight days, let's hear it for 'the change'.

Not all women experience all the following adjustments to the same degree. Some you may not even notice. Others will be more upsetting to you than they are to the next woman. The main thing to remember about these physical developments is that, if they cause you pain, there is usually something you can do or take to relieve the discomfort.

Breasts

Breasts may lose their fullness and firmness as less oestrogen stimulates the tissue. After the menopause, breasts of thin women often become smaller and flatter and those of obese women become pendulous. Loss of elasticity in some ligaments aggravates the tendency of breasts to droop and the nipples become smaller and flatter and may lose their erectile properties.

The breast

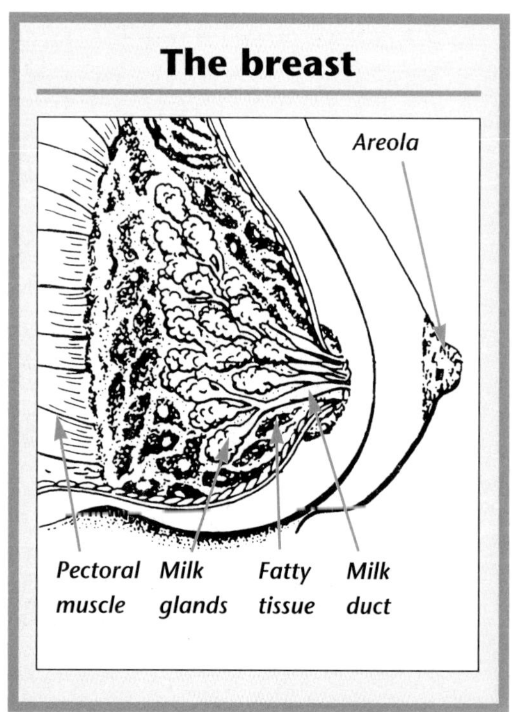

Examining your breasts

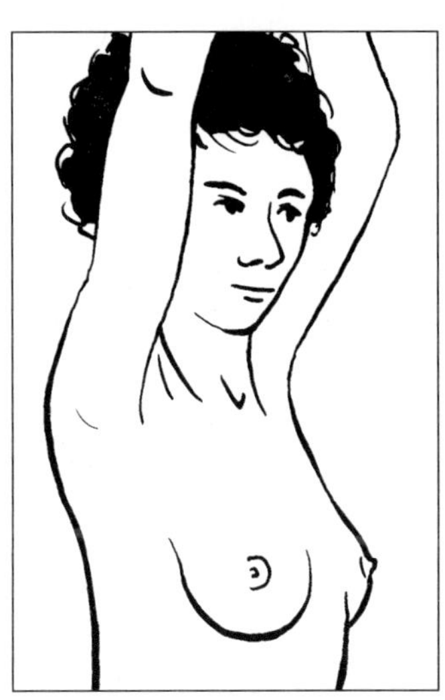

1 Standing in front of a mirror, look at your breasts and position of the nipples. 2 Raise your arms and look for any changes in the breasts' shape and size. Turn to look at them sideways as well. 3 Lie down with your arms at your sides and gently press one breast in a circular movement. Place your other arm above your head and check underneath and outside the breast and in the armpit for lumps. Repeat with the other breast. If you detect a lump or anything unusual, don't be afraid to consult your doctor immediately.

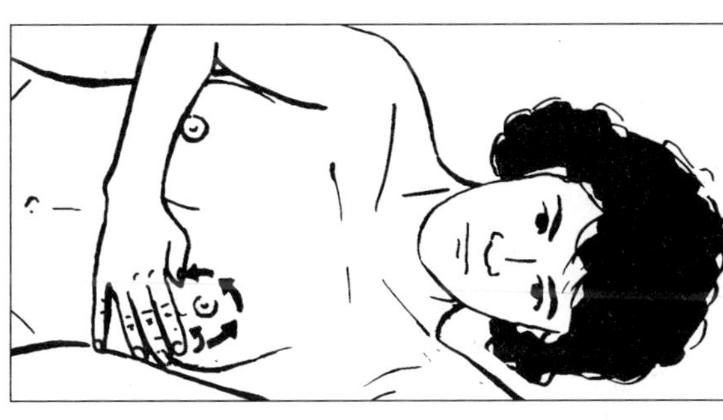

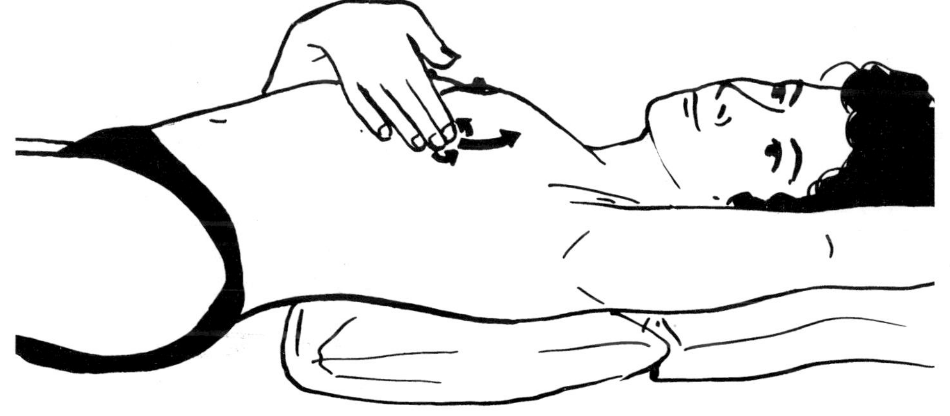

Taking an oestrogen supplement may stave off some of the above changes but you can also help yourself by doing a few simple exercises every day.

Ovaries

The ovaries are the most powerful glands in a woman's body, controlling the reproductive system. The difference between one woman and another – and how easy/difficult her menopause is – depends on the amount of hormone produced by the ovaries because they affect all our tissues. Ideally you should have a regular pelvic examination to make sure your ovaries are sound. Any swelling or pain in the lower abdomen where the ovaries are, needs to be reported immediately because it could signal cancer. A few incidents of ovarian cancer appear to be hereditary and there seems to be a link between it and breast cancer.

Women who lose ovarian function at an early age are more at risk of heart disease and osteoporosis. For instance, women who had been oophorectomised (their ovaries removed) at the age of 30 were found, 20 years later, to have bone mass loss in spine, hip and wrist comparable to 70-year-old women who underwent natural menopause at the age of 50 years.

The ovaries

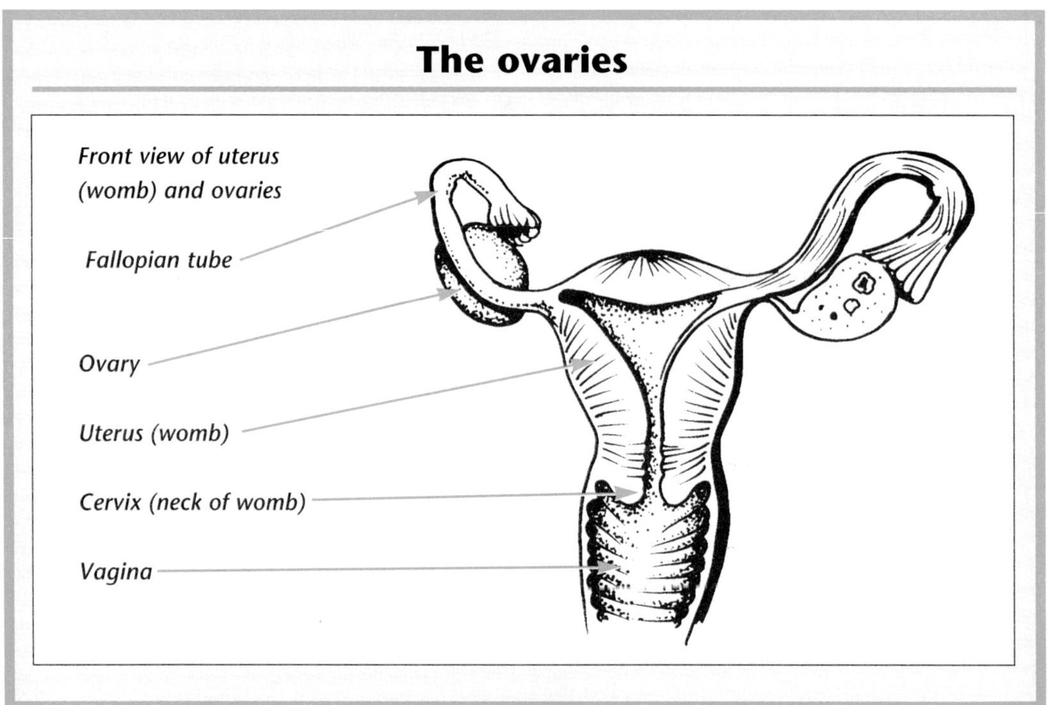

Uterus and cervix

The uterus, or womb, has thick, muscular walls and its cavity is normally just a slit but, of course, capable of enormous expansion during pregnancy. The cervix, the narrower neck end which goes down into the vagina, is where smear tests for cancer and other abnormalities are taken from. In time the cervix shrinks and retracts and sometimes becomes flush with the vaginal wall. Early in the climacteric there is a gradual diminution of the mucous when it becomes sparse and thin.

The cavity of the uterus is lined with a special tissue called the endometrium which oestrogen stimulates during the first half of

The uterus and cervix

Womb
Normal cervix
Vagina

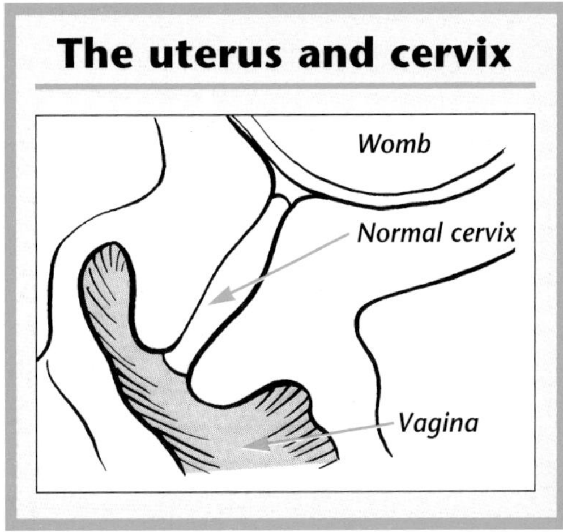

Female pelvic area

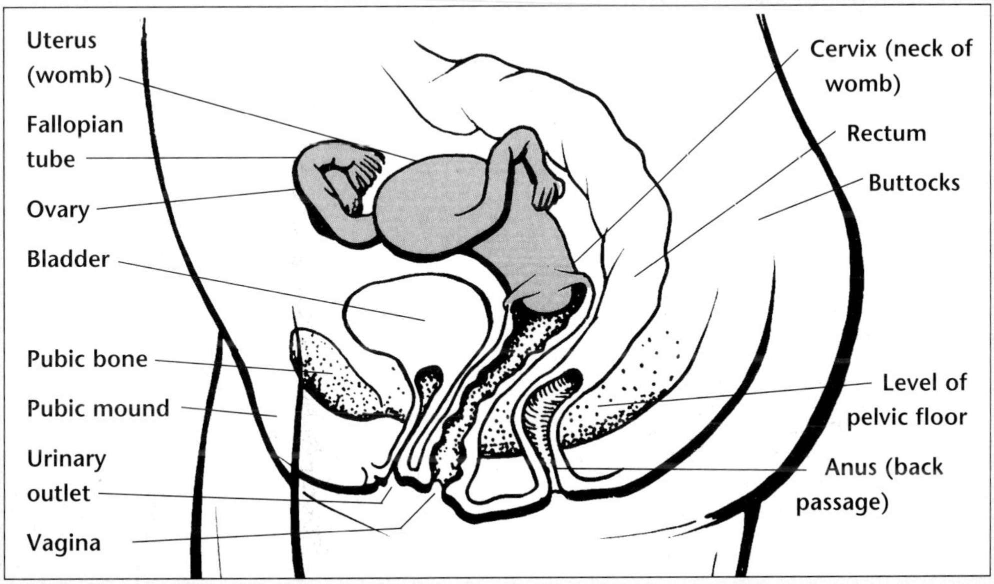

Uterus (womb)
Fallopian tube
Ovary
Bladder
Pubic bone
Pubic mound
Urinary outlet
Vagina
Cervix (neck of womb)
Rectum
Buttocks
Level of pelvic floor
Anus (back passage)

Endometriosis

This refers to the growth of small patches of endometrium (or lining of the womb) at other sites in the body. These are usually around the womb and the ovaries or can very occasionally occur elsewhere in the body. Each time you have a period these small areas of misplaced tissue bleed in just the same way, causing a great deal of pain because the blood cannot get out. Endometriosis is not cancer but can cause many other problems such as:

- Internal bleeding.
- Inflammation and scar tissue pain.
- Adhesions of internal organs.
- Infertility.

Adenomyosis is the name given to endometriosis which becomes dispersed in sheets throughout the muscle layers of the womb causing a tender enlarged uterus. It is difficult to diagnose prior to hysterectomy.

Endometrial hyperplasia refers to an overgrowth of the lining of the womb caused by hormone imbalance. Not all hyperplasia is dangerous. Very often, if treated, it regresses and becomes normal. In one per cent of all cases the changes can progress to cancer so it is a condition which needs to be watched carefully by examining small samples from the lining of the womb at regular intervals.

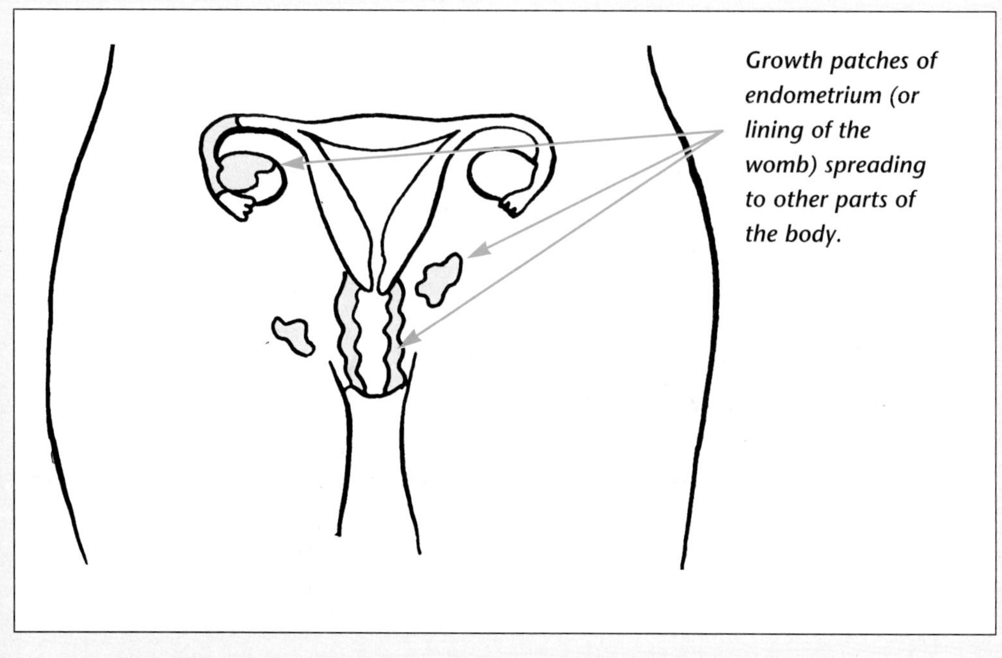

the cycle making it thicker and more muscular. Progesterone is added during the second phase of the cycle when the endometrium gets thicker still and becomes rich in blood vessels. It is shreds of endometrium which, when they are not disgorged properly, can drift off, glueing one pelvic organ to another, causing a particularly painful condition called endometriosis.

Prolapse

The womb gets smaller after the menopause and, like the ovaries, can be quite tiny in old age. The supporting ligaments and tissues become weaker as the menopause approaches, the dwindling supply of oestrogen reducing their elasticity and firmness. This can cause what is known as a prolapse – literally slipping forwards or downwards. There is a much higher incidence of this in women who have had children.

In extreme cases the womb can slip right outside the vagina but most often what happens is it drops just a fraction but it may still be painful, uncomfortable or potentially dangerous so surgery has to be performed. No surgery is simple in my view but operations to correct a prolapse are commonplace, relatively painless and usually very successful.

How to tell if you have a prolapse

- A sensation of something dropping down your vagina.
- Feeling there is an obstruction during intercourse.
- Difficulty passing faeces.
- Difficulty trying to pass water.
- Backache which you don't normally suffer from.

Prolapse – before and after

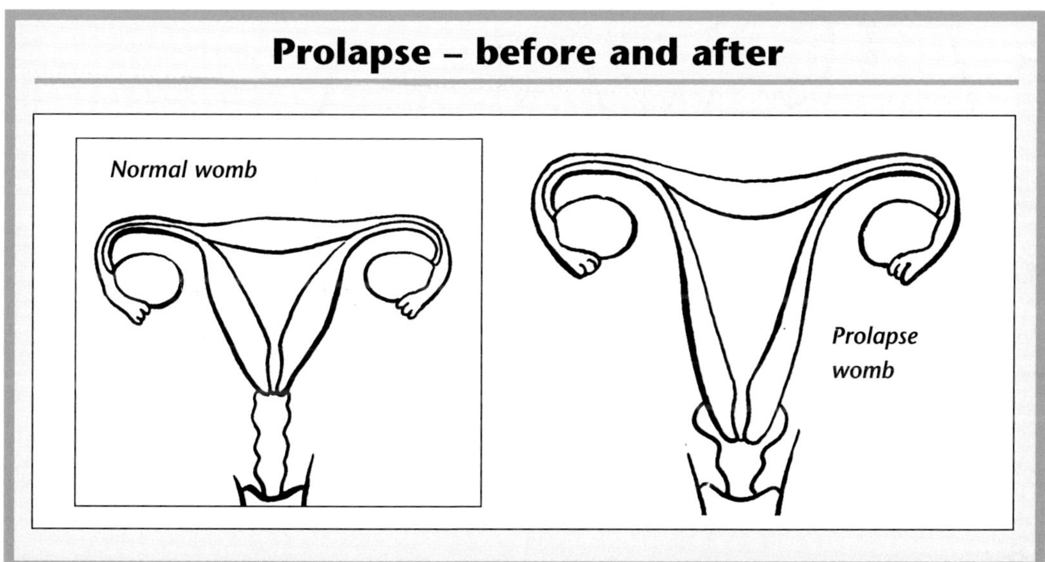

Help, what is happening to me?

Vagina

The vagina is a hollow muscular tube about nine centimetres long leading to the womb. It is lined by folds of skin capable of considerable expansion. The medical term 'vaginal atrophy' sounds particularly negative and although changes potentially for the worse do occur to this vital part of our anatomy, you do not have to lie back and do nothing. The regular production of oestrogen keeps the vaginal wall strong and elastic, producing enough vaginal fluids to keep the area moist. So, obviously, once the supply of oestrogen dries up, so does the vagina.

Normally a process of cell regeneration occurs which produces lactic acid. This is nature's way of keeping the environment of the vagina free of infection from outside contamination. After the menopause the lining skin of the vagina becomes thin so this process of lactic acid production may be interfered with in which case inflammation, or 'vaginitis', can occur. A vaginal irritation can be merely uncomfortable or extremely painful in which case you ought to consult your doctor, especially if it goes on for any length of time or recurs frequently

For women who are still sexually active, often the worst effects of the menopause is dryness of the vagina. It is essential to talk to your partner about this as it will affect him too. If he has to force his way into a dry passage he could 'burn' his penis which will turn you both off sex. Most women use a lubricant which is often all that is required. A low-dose oestrogen cream on prescription will not only increase the amount of oestrogen acting locally on the vaginal wall,

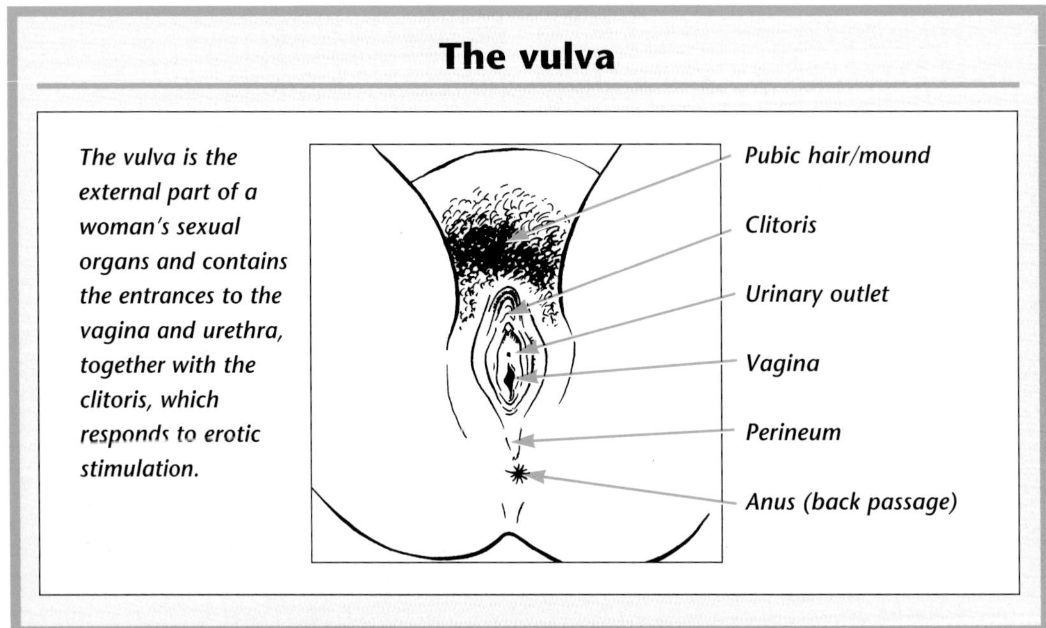

but it will also be absorbed into the blood stream. This combination helps to thicken the tissues of the vagina which in turn will help it to produce more mucous so it becomes properly lubricated 'naturally'.

Paradoxically, the menopause often brings with it a welcome boost to women's sex lives. They no longer fear pregnancy and they have the confidence to talk about what arouses them. Children are not at home to interrupt and they can go to bed at unconventional times. Once you start talking to women about their postmenopausal sex life you begin to realise what a boon rather than a bother the whole business can be.

The other good news is that according to some studies, the more sexually active you are into middle-age, the more you help to preserve vaginal function after the menopause. Intercourse stimulates the vagina so, after all, there is a satisfactory equation to be addressed:

- The menopause = dry vagina.
- Dry vagina = difficult sex.
- Difficult sex = no sex **OR**
- Stimulation = moist vagina.
- Moist vagina = satisfactory sex.
- Satisfactory sex = good sex.
- Good sex = more sex.

Vulva

The vulva is several structures which surround the entrance to the vagina and consists of a number of separate entities.

The labia majora are two large folds of skin filled with fat and containing hair follicles and sweat glands. They vary in size, becoming smaller after the menopause. In front they merge into the pad of fat which lies over the pubic bone. This is known as the mons pubis, or Mount of Venus, and is covered by skin and hairs.

The labia minora, or inner lips, become almost non-existent after the menopause and many women experience itchiness because the vaginal orifice, being less protected by its 'lips,' is more exposed to infection.

The clitoris also becomes smaller as the reproductive epoch fades but it still responds to stimulation so there is no reason why you should not enjoy an orgasm, although as you get older the contractions usually decrease.

Sexual intercourse and childbirth produce a number of changes to the area between the vagina and anus: it may have been stretched or torn and the vaginal orifice can become wider. Generally the condition of the vulva can be improved by oestrogen or corticosteroid therapy.

Hysterectomy

A hysterectomy is an operation to remove the womb. The name comes from the Greek words 'hustera' for womb, and 'ektome' for excision. It sometimes also involves the removal of one or both ovaries and one or both fallopian tubes.

There are two ways of performing a hysterectomy, depending on the medical conditions, and you should ask your surgeon which one is being planned for you and

Help, what is happening to me?

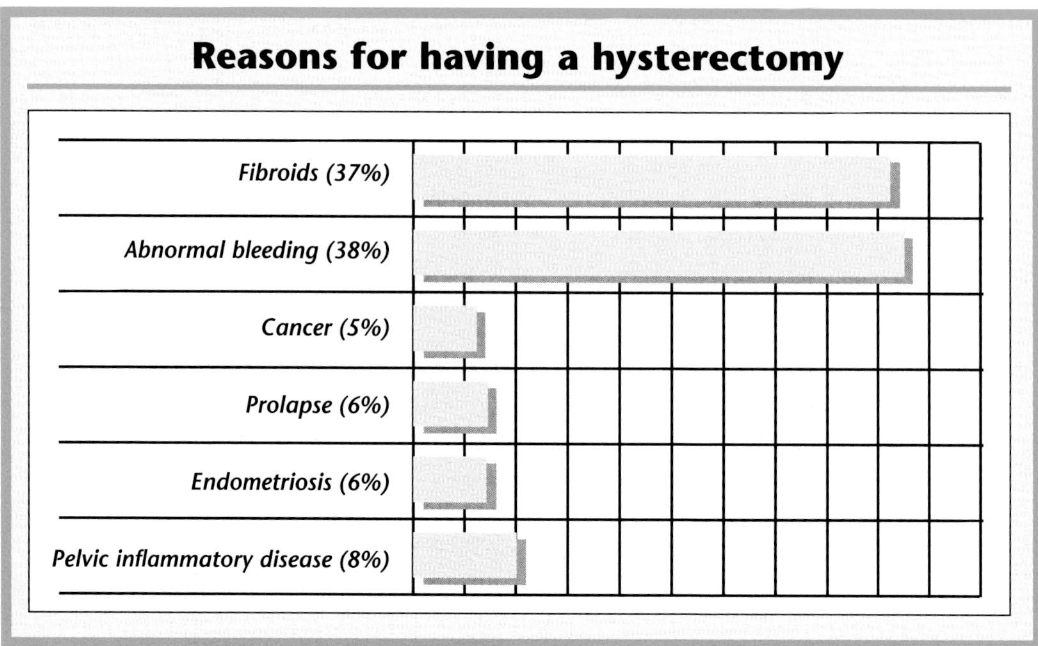

why. An abdominal hysterectomy is performed through an opening in the lower abdominal wall and leaves a thin scar along the bikini line. A vaginal hysterectomy leaves no external scars but may not be suitable.

Heavy bleeding, a not uncommon occurrence during the menopause, is the reason why thirty-eight per cent of hysterectomies are performed. The next significant factor is fibroids which accounts for thirty-seven per cent of the women who opt for this operation. Other causes, although much less significant in terms of numbers – between eight and five per cent – are pelvic inflammatory disease, endometriosis, prolapse and cancer. What constitutes heavy bleeding is really a matter for each individual woman to decide but most can tell the difference between what they have experienced during approximately forty years of periods and the onset of an unaccustomed flood. It is then up to each woman to make the decision about how to tackle the problem. Some opt straightaway for a hysterectomy but others prefer to endure the discomfort and inconvenience until it eventually stops but it is a decision which ought to be made with the advice of a gynaecologist.

Losing a lot of blood can cause iron deficiency anaemia, besides making you feel incredibly unwell or even totally incapacitated. On the other hand, many women are still reluctant to have a hysterectomy on the grounds they feel they will be less of a woman afterwards although those who do have one generally report never having felt better. And it doesn't have any detrimental effect on their love life. If anything, they report the reverse because their pain and anxieties are removed.

Fibroids

Fibroids are often referred to in fruity terms by doctors – the size of a grape, plum, orange, – etc. which is as good a way as any for explaining how big or small they are to the laywoman. A fibroid is a mass of muscle tissue that can grow at various sites within and around the womb. It is not a cancer. However, fibroids can grow very large and cause pain and heavy bleeding. They can also become a medical emergency if they suddenly twist themselves or cause blockages. If they are small they cause few, if any, problems and may go unnoticed. But the larger they become, the more problems they can cause including:

- Abdominal swelling.
- Pelvic and back pain.
- Infertility.
- Heavy and irregular bleeding.
- Painful periods.
- Constipation.
- Pressure on the bladder.

Pelvic inflammatory disease

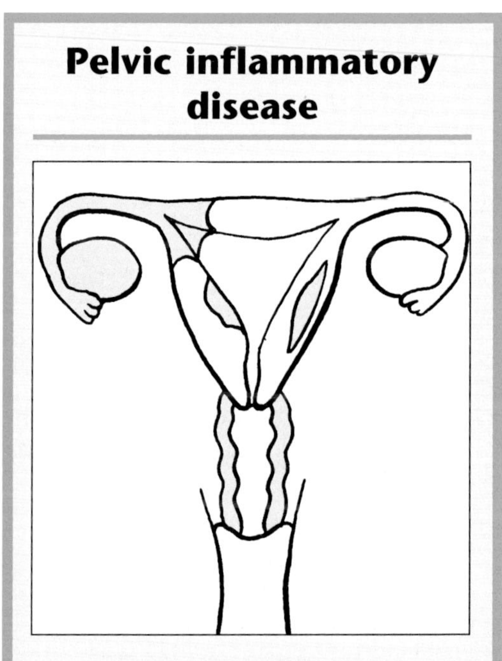

Pelvic inflammatory disease

Pelvic inflammatory diseases can be caused by sexual intercourse, intra-uterine contraceptive devices, following childbirth or abortion, or can be spread via the bloodstream from infections elsewhere in the body. They can affect the ovaries, fallopian tubes or uterus, and chronic inflammation associated with longstanding infections can cause:

- Vague feelings of illness.
- Pain.
- Dyspareunia (pain associated with intercourse).
- Infertility from blockage of the fallopian tubes.
- Pungent vaginal discharge.
- Internal scarring.
- Adhesions (sticking together) of pelvic organs.

If caught early, pelvic inflammatory disease can be treated with antibiotics but if it is very severe, then a hysterectomy and removal of the damaged tissue may be the only solution.

The womb, as mentioned earlier, in spite of being able to stretch to accommodate a very large baby, is really quite small: about the

Position of uterus

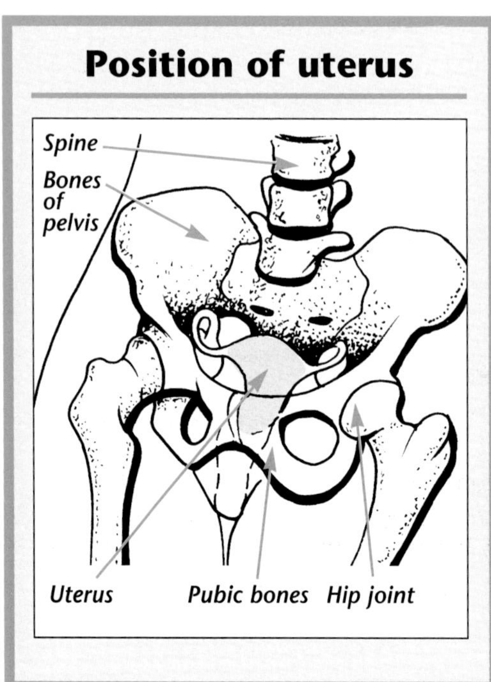

size of a large pear. The ovaries are almond-shaped and only about one and a half inches long so, even if they are all removed, there is not a huge empty space left behind. If they have been enlarged by fibroids or disease, then the surrounding organs will have been pushed out of place. Once removed, the bladder, bowel and intestines soon move around to take up the space. And the gap at the top end of the vagina where the cervix used to be will be closed off by stitches.

Total hysterectomy

Total hysterectomy is a bit of a misnomer because, although the womb is removed, the ovaries are not. Besides the elimination of a bleeding problem, a total hysterectomy also removes the possibility of fibroids or a prolapse occurring later. It also removes the necessity for cervical smear tests since the cervix is gone. A few gynaecologists still perform a subtotal hysterectomy when the main body of the womb is removed but the neck of the womb, the cervix, which is a potential site for cancer, is left behind. You should query why this, though a relatively quick and easy operation, is the preferred option.

Hysterectomy with oophorectomy

Hysterectomy with oophorectomy (removal of the ovaries) is, in the view of the vast majority of gynaecologists, the preferred option for postmenopausal women. Obviously, once the womb is removed, you will have no more periods but if the ovaries are still in place they will still be susceptible to developing cysts, pain or even cancer. They do carry on producing the hormones oestrogen and progesterone in their usual monthly cycle. However, there is evidence that the production of hormones declines markedly within a year or two of a hysterectomy in some women. The argument, therefore, is that you may as well get rid of them while you are having a hysterectomy. A prophylactic (preventive) oophorectomy may be the sensible course but it is up to you to decide.

Total hysterectomy with bilateral salpingo-oophorectomy

When the womb, cervix, fallopian tubes and ovaries are all removed, it is called a total hysterectomy with bilateral salpingo-oophorectomy. This operation is sometimes chosen, particularly for women with conditions which affect all the tissues involved: large fibroids, cancer, extensive endometriosis or longstanding pelvic infection.

Radical hysterectomy involves all the above plus the removal of the top of the vagina, together with surrounding fatty tissue and lymph glands in the pelvis. It is an extensive operation usually performed for early cancer of the cervix or of the endometrium, the lining of the womb, which aims to remove any local spread of the disease.

Types of hysterectomy

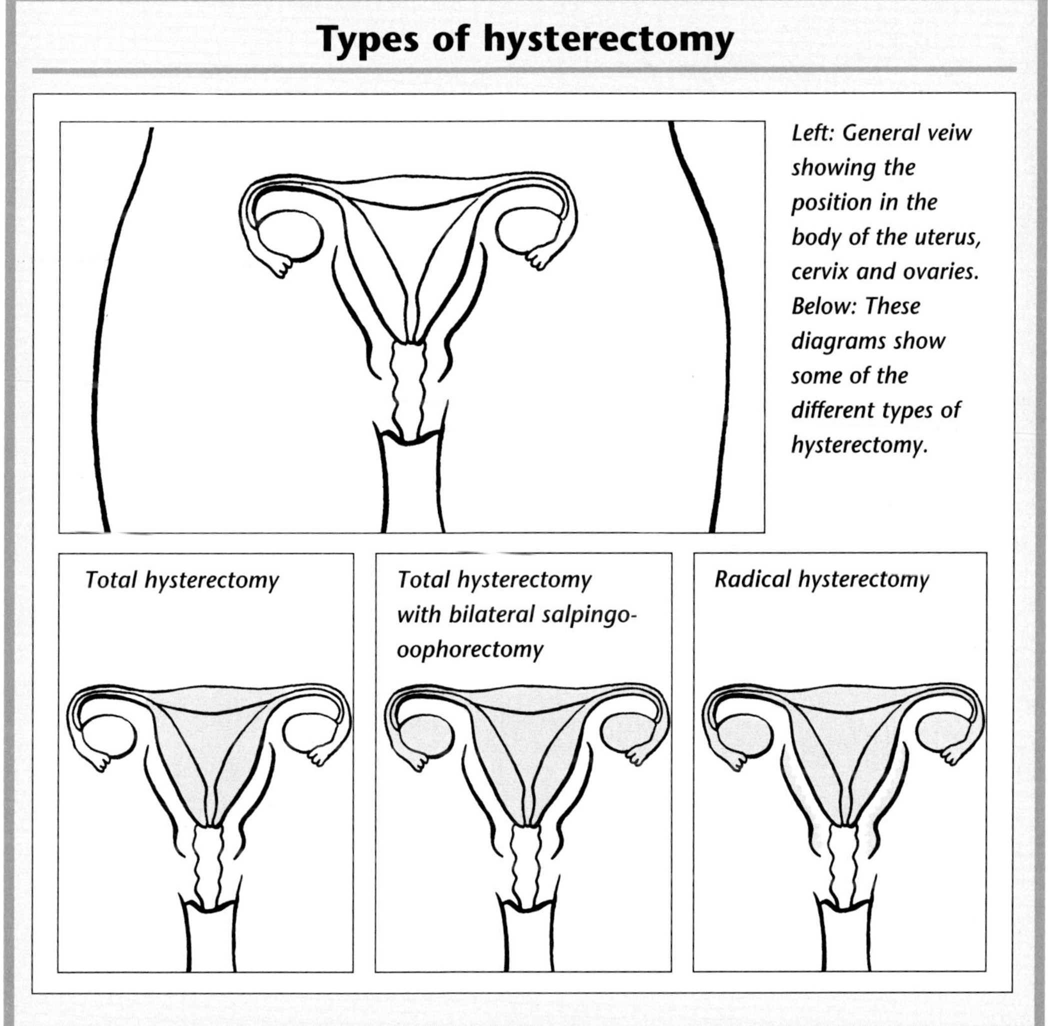

Left: General veiw showing the position in the body of the uterus, cervix and ovaries. Below: These diagrams show some of the different types of hysterectomy.

Getting out of bed after a hysterectomy

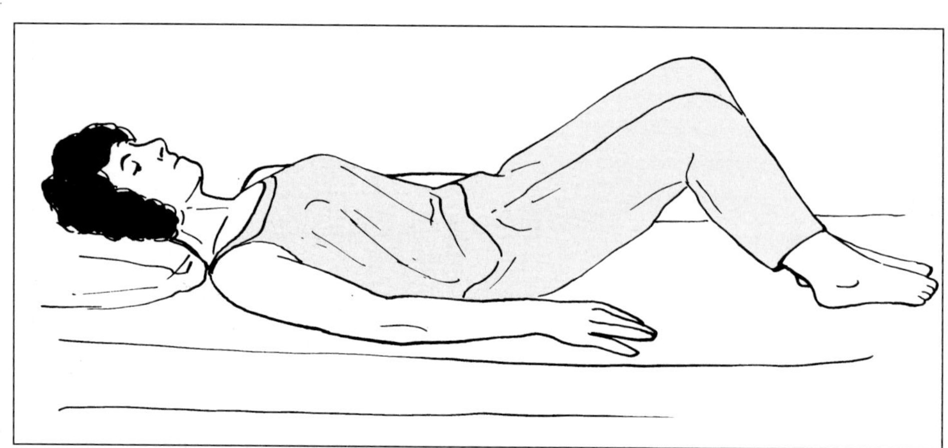

It is important not to exert any strain on the pelvic area when getting out of bed. Slide your feet up towards your bottom to bend your knees. With knees bent, roll onto your side and push down with hands or elbows. Slowly swing your legs over the edge of the bed and raise yourself up into a sitting position.

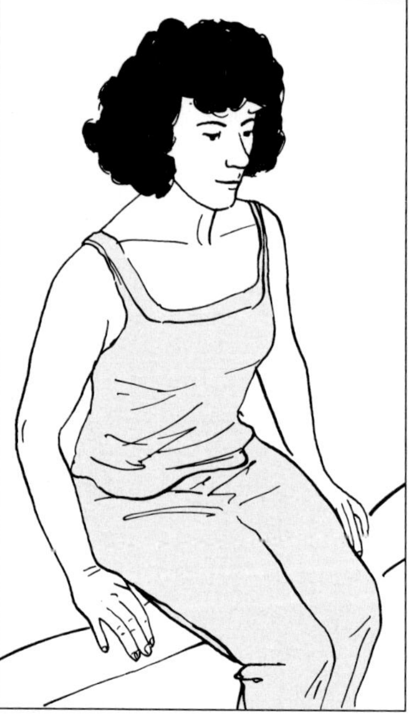

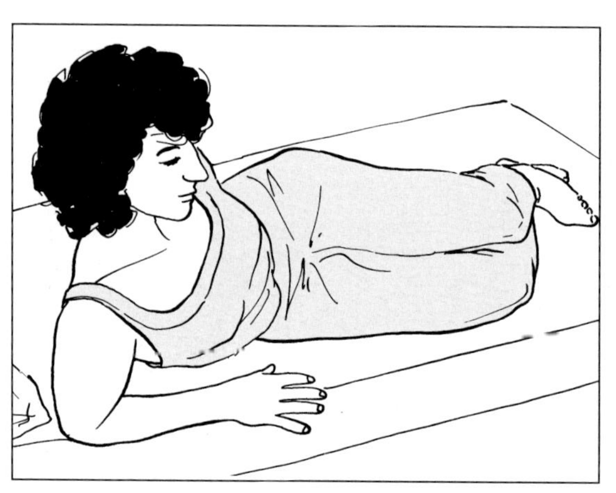

Exercises after a hysterectomy

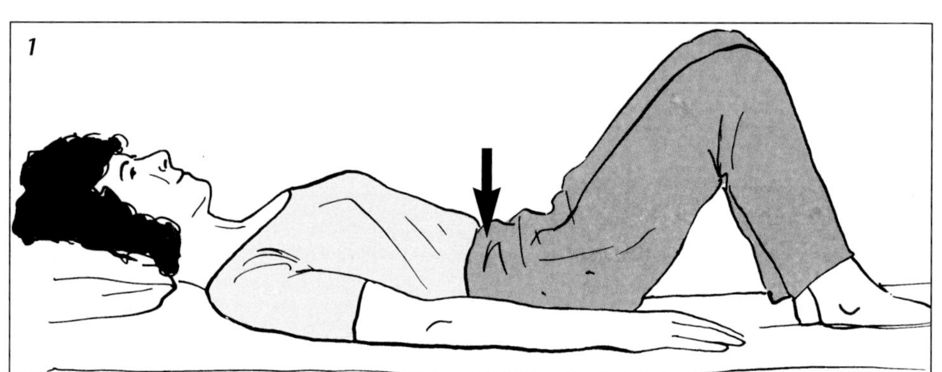
1

These exercises will help tighten up tummy muscles.

***1** Lie with knees bent and arms at sides. Pull in your tummy muscles and hold for a count of 4. Relax and repeat 5 times.*

***2** With a cushion to support your head, lie down with knees bent.*

***3** With hands resting on thighs, slowly lift your head. Look at your knees, tucking your chin into your chest. Hold for a count of 4, lower and then repeat 5 times.*

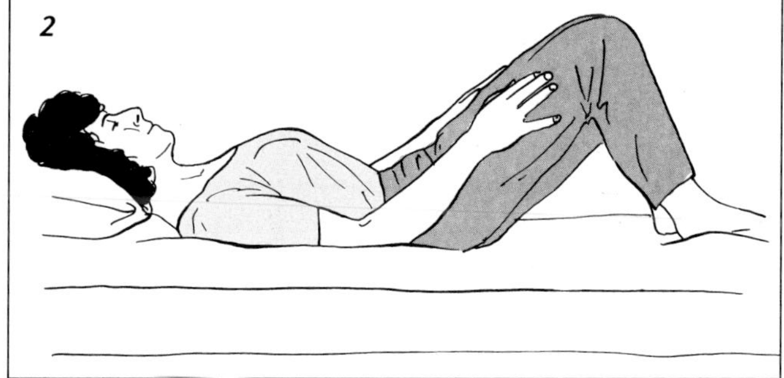
2

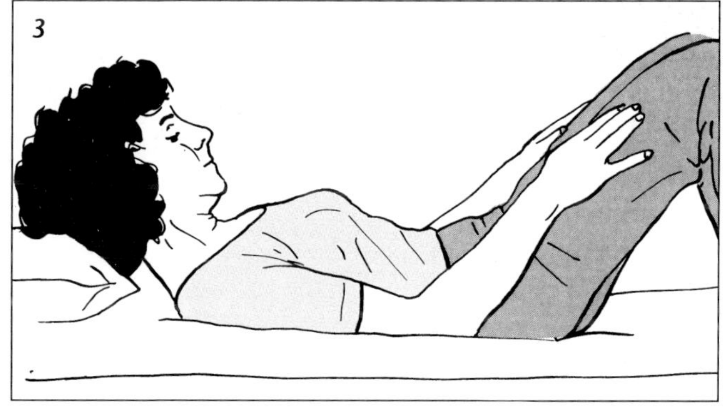
3

Chapter three

The ageing heart and old bones

Heart disease and osteoporosis are the two demons which haunt the menopause. There is no argument about how much they cost in terms of lives lost or ruined because of them but there is a great deal of controversy about the best way to avoid them. Basically the difference is between chemical interference and diet. You either believe the first will do you an enormous amount of good while the second is also quite important, or you think the first will do you nothing but harm and the second is the key to staving off both conditions.

My own view is somewhere in between. If you can tailor your food requirements to suit your body's needs then natural treatment has to be the best way to tackle anything. These killers sneak up on us; there are usually no handy warning signals as we approach the menopause, but if you have a family history or personal medical condition which suggests you might be vulnerable to a heart attack, stroke or osteoporosis, it seems sensible to take advantage of all that modern medicine has to offer.

Heart disease

Ischaemic heart disease (IHD) and stroke are the commonest causes of death in both men and women in Great Britain. IHD is six times lower in women than in men between the ages of 35-44 but only two times lower by the age of 50. The reason is believed to be because of the menopause. Before that women are protected by their oestrogen: when that drops so their blood cholesterol and triglyceride rise and with it the risk of a heart attack. This is why, if a woman has to have a hysterectomy, especially if she is still young, she should not have her ovaries removed if they are healthy because their

Risk factors

- Premature menopause.
- Hereditary high level of cholesterol.
- A family history of heart disease.
- Hypertension.
- Diabetes.
- Cigarette smoking.
- Obesity.
- Type A personality (a stress junkie).
- A diet high in saturated fat.

oestrogen production is vital to her general health. Oestrogen also relaxes the muscle walls of blood vessels causing dilatation of vessels and improved circulation. This may in part explain the lower incidence of coronary thrombosis in women.

Diet and the heart

Diet plays a major part in heart disease and it makes sense, if women are at greater risk during and after the menopause, to pay particular attention to your eating habits once the menopause has started. Advice about what to eat is in Part Three but the crucial thing to take on board is that your metabolism slows down as you get older, so your digestive system cannot cope with as much food as it once did but you still require the same amount of nutrients.

Diet and osteoporosis

Eating a healthy, balanced diet with an adequate amount of calcium helps to build healthy bones and prevent osteoporosis. Calcium is important throughout a woman's life: particularly during childhood, adolescence and pregnancy, when breastfeeding and in later life.

The best sources of calcium are cheese, milk and yogurt. Weight watchers can still get as much calcium from low-fat alternatives, e.g. skimmed milk. Other sources of calcium are sardines and whitebait (fish where you eat the bones), nuts, seeds and green vegetables.

Osteoporosis

Osteoporosis is a serious bone disease which affects almost half the female population by the time they are 80. It is ten times more common among women than men and the most common cause is oestrogen deficiency which occurs when ovaries fail naturally or after surgery. Of the 52,000 women in the UK who suffered hip fractures in 1990, one in five died as a result from associated illnesses like pneumonia, blood clots, infection or stroke. Half will never be able to lead independent lives again: large numbers require long-term nursing care and/or sheltered accommodation. The financial cost of osteoporotic fractures is enormous yet it is a disease which is preventable and is probably the most significant reason why hormone replacement therapy is growing in popularity, in spite of the reluctance on the part of some doctors to prescribe it. Osteoporosis is the medical term which in laywoman's language means brittle bones.

The ageing heart and old bones

Bones lose some of their density, they become more porous and brittle and therefore break more easily. Besides fractures, the most obvious outward sign of bones deteriorating is 'dowager's hump': a bent or stooped back which is the result of vertebrae collapsing or being wedged together.

Unfortunately, osteoporosis proceeds by stealth. To detect it you need a bone density scan which is not readily available on the NHS in the UK and is quite costly to have done privately. Peak bone mass, achieved in your mid to late thirties, is largely genetically determined, hence the importance of a family history of osteoporosis in predicting fracture risk in an individual. Lifestyle factors can also affect bone mass. Heavy smoking and more than two alcoholic drinks a day reduce hip bone density by a substantial amount in women in their late 40s. Bone loss also appears to be accelerate more after an early hysterectomy then after natural menopause, but the over-riding factor is lack of oestrogen which is why a hormone replacement is recommended now by most doctors for menopausal women to prevent this disease.

Bone density

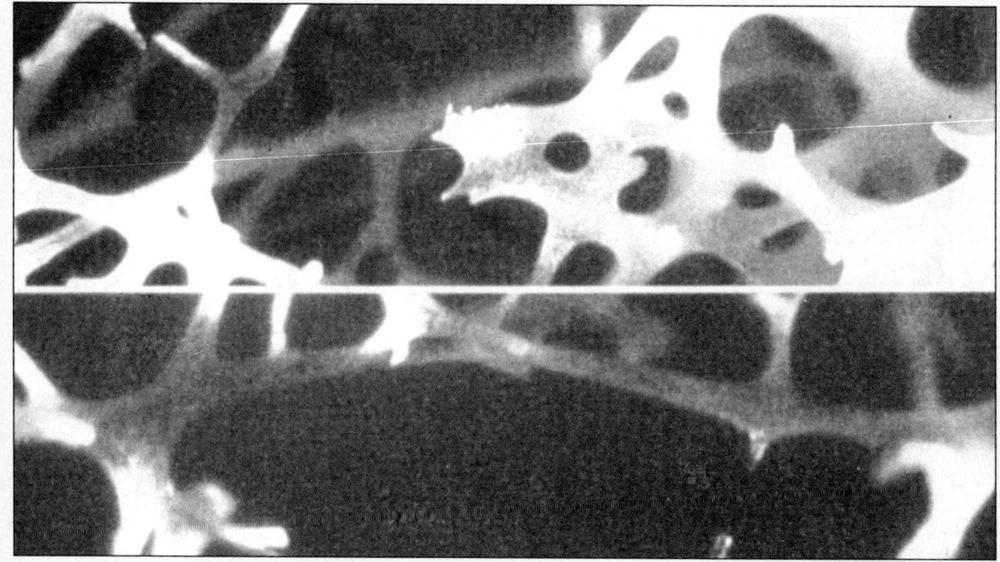

These micrograph pictures show the appearance of normal bone (top) and osteoporotic bone (below). The interior of normal bone is filled with cells, but in osteoporosis their density decreases. Thus the bones become less strong and more brittle, and are liable to fracture easily.

Spinal problems due to osteoporosis

The spine is made up of a long series of small bones called vertebrae. Healed vertebral fractures become compressed (flattened) or may mend in a wedge shape. Over a period of time, compression fractures can cause the spine to begin collapsing, leading to pain, a loss of height and eventually stooped posture. Even one compression fracture weakens the spine. Osteoporosis often leads to multiple compression fractures that will permanently change the strength and shape of the spine. This makes it very important to diagnose the disease as early as possible.

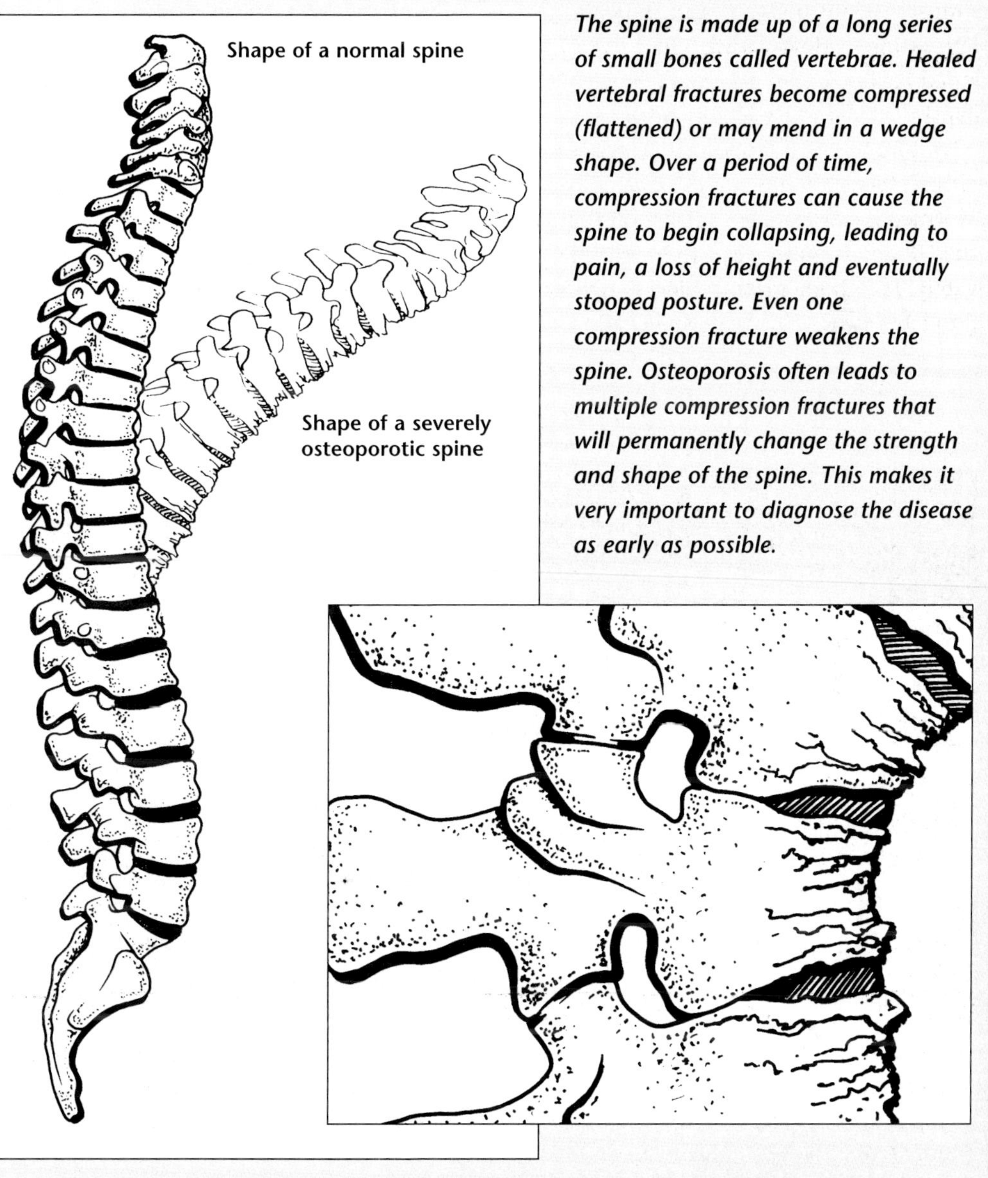

The ageing heart and old bones

Premature osteoporosis

The onset of premature osteoporosis developing is increased by the following:

- Failure of the ovaries to develop.
- Too much prolactin in the blood.
- Amenorrhoea (no periods) caused by excessive physical exercise, e.g. in women athletes and dancers.
- Amenorrhoea caused by drugs used in the treatment of endometriosis.
- Premature menopause (before 45).
- Osteoporosis in a close female relative.
- High alcohol intake.
- Cigarette smoking.
- Low body mass (small stature and small bones).
- Inadequate calcium intake when young.
- Infertility.
- Sedentary lifestyle.
- Long-term use of corticosteroids.
- Anorexia nervosa.
- Exceptional intake of caffeine.
- Steroids for arthritis, asthma or ulcerative colitis.
- Some drugs used in the treatment of epilepsy.

However, it needs to be said that patients with multiple risk factors have been shown to have satisfactory skeletal preservation in both the spine and hip and conversely, patients with no risk factor have demonstrated considerable bone density loss within two years of the menopause.

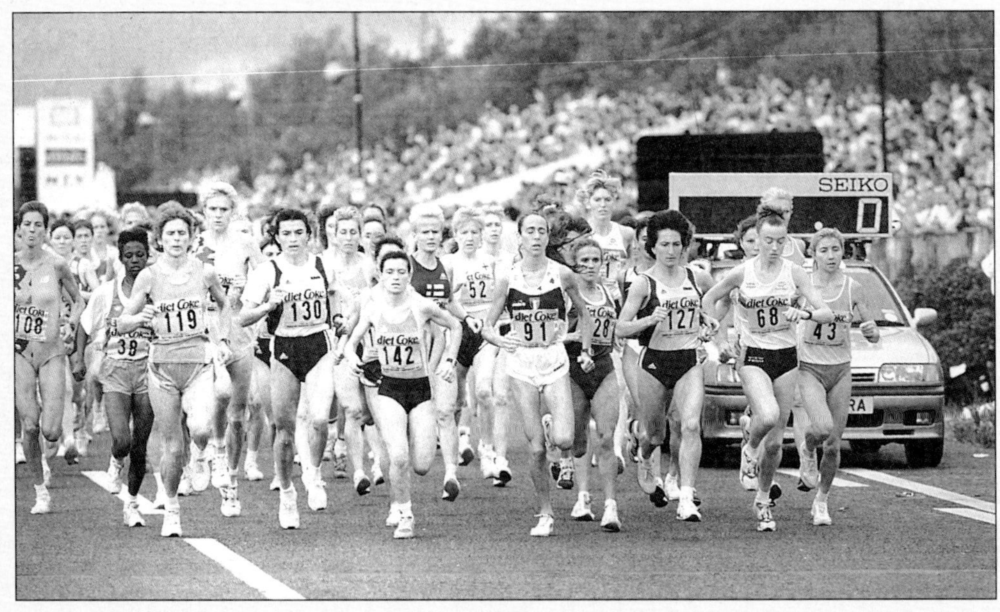

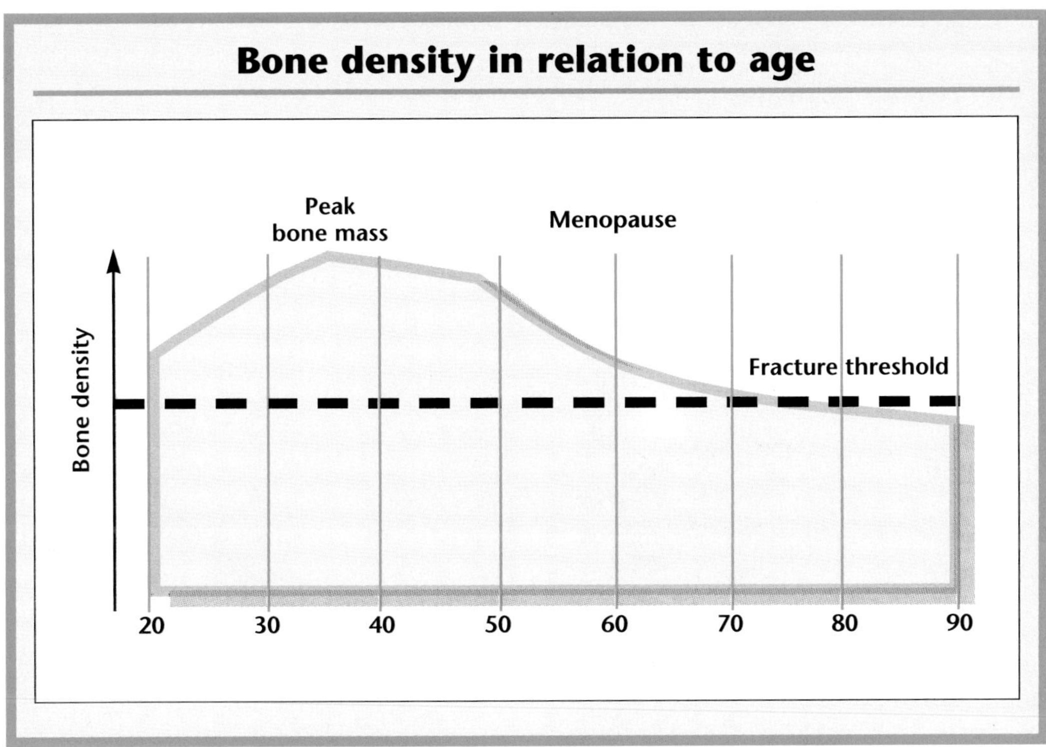

Treatments for osteoporosis

These depend on the woman's age, previous medical history and the degree to which she is affected by osteoporosis. Hormone replacement therapy (HRT) is often prescribed for women under 65 years. This is described in detail later in the book. It is a safe and effective method of preventing further bone loss, and is available in the form of pills, patches and implants.

Advantages of HRT

It has been shown that women who take HRT for at least five years, starting soon after menopause, reduce their fracture risk by approximately 60 per cent. Scientific studies have also shown that HRT reduces the risk of heart disease, as well as eliminating such menopausal symptoms as headaches and hot flushes. Therefore HRT is now recommended by many doctors.

Chapter four

All in the mind

Probably the most irritating remark in the menopause lexicon is "snap out of it". We suffer incredible, sometimes terrifying, switches in mood and that is the response we get. Is it any wonder we are sometimes driven mad? There are many circumstances which can affect our mood. Obviously someone treating us badly is the main one but because arriving at the menopause age is also a time for taking stock, the prospects before us can be quite daunting. You gaze into the past and wonder what you have done with your life and you look into the future and wonder what you are going to do with the rest of it.

But there is no doubt, too, that our hormones as well as our mineral and protein balance affect our mood. Many doctors believe that for our mental health, zinc and copper influences need to be equal and research has revealed that some schizophrenics have exceptionally high blood copper levels. Shortage of vitamin B6 may also lead to lack of mental balance.

Oestrogen, often called the feel-good hormone, is sometimes given to relieve depression but it should not be regarded as a general panacea.

Sleeplessness

Insomnia may begin to be a problem during the menopause. Obviously night sweats and needing to empty your bladder more often are two common causes. Some women find it hard to get back to sleep and if they have a partner it can develop into rows because he will lose sleep too. There are a number of things you can do before resorting to the spare bedroom:

- Never eat after seven in the evening.
- Don't have anything to drink later than that either.
- Take more exercise. A walk, run, swim (especially aquarobics) will help you to sleep.

What you should not do is take sleeping pills. They can become addictive, they give totally distorted sleep patterns and may make you feel quite groggy in the morning. In the self-help section there are other suggestions to overcome sleeplessness which I hope you will try before resorting to drugs.

Remember, too, that your sleep pattern often changes with age: the body requires less. So it is not something you should waste too much time worrying about unless it seriously undermines your ability to function the following day. Worrying exacerbates most problems. Is it possible, for instance, to sneak forty winks during the day? Don't be ashamed: I know a very high-powered executive who, although it is extremely difficult to organise, has to do it. There are many relaxation tapes available now which are extremely good and helpful. You can learn how to meditate – an increasingly popular way of relaxing.

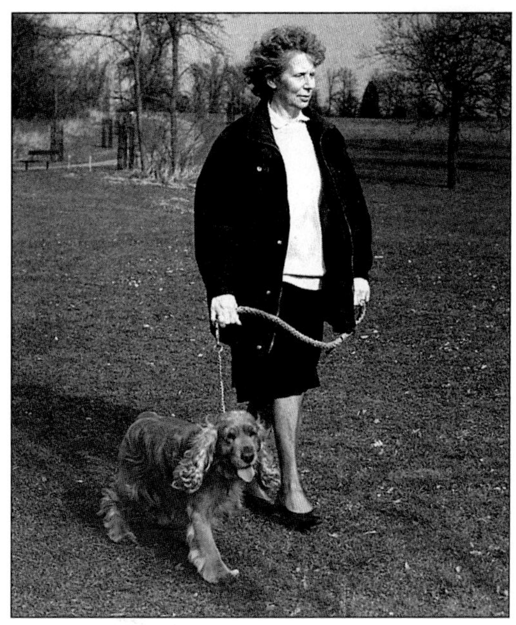

If you suffer from insomnia, taking regular exercise will help you to sleep as well as improving your general health and well-being and keeping you fit. Try to exercise several times a week, even if it's only going for a walk.

Tired all the time

Clearly, if you are having trouble sleeping, you may be tired all the time (TATT) but this does not necessarily have to be caused by insomnia. Many middle-aged women start noticing they are lacking in energy and blame the menopause although there may be other reasons. Doing too much can be one. When I talk to groups of women about their health I always start by asking them, "What did you do today?" It is quite staggering the amount of work women get through.

Being exhausted is not a pre-condition of the menopause but it can be a warning signal from your body to give it a break so if you are suffering from TATT I suggest you try and put some of the following into practice:

- ME time. It is essential to put aside at least an hour every day to doing things just for yourself. Read a book or paint your nails; don't just watch television because you won't feel you have lavished time on yourself and that is the feeling you need to experience.
- Check your diet. There are suggestions in Chapter Seven for things you can eat to give yourself an energy boost.
- Lose weight. While carrying excess baggage around may not have mattered so much when you were younger, now your muscles, joints etc. are not so strong it has more serious consequences.

All in the mind

Mood swings

For women going through the menopause there are certain hormonal modifications which, try as they might, are bound to affect their mood. Unfortunately, because of the timing, other major changes can also have a bearing on your mood and it is sometimes difficult to unravel what it is, exactly, that is causing your distress.

- Is it because your adolescent children are giving you a hard time?
- Is it because they are going off to university and you are suffering from the notorious 'empty nest syndrome'?
- Is it because you are going through a divorce?
- Is it because you have been in the same job now for twenty years?
- Is it because your finances are shaky?
- Is it because the prospect of having to care for an elderly relative is looming?

All these are legitimate causes for anxiety so it is hardly surprising if they affect your mood. How do you tell when the feeling of depression is caused by a life event and when it is hormonal? The answer is you can't but it is useful to remember that it may not be "all in the mind". The old-fashioned advice to "snap out of it" which many women were given when they complained of feeling low will not wash today. So, what can you do?

Keep a mood diary. Record how fed up you feel, on a scale of 0-5; what happened before you felt so stressed. Make a note of anything or anyone who has upset you.

Cut down on alcohol because nothing distorts the emotions like too much to drink, and check your diet. There are many foods which cause mood swings, like chocolate and cheese. Or you could be lacking in a vital vitamin or mineral.

Apologise to your children if they have borne the brunt of your grumpiness. They may even admit they are part of the problem and be more helpful and understanding which will make you feel better. In the self-help section I will be talking about exercise which can swing a blue mood into a sunny one.

Be kind to yourself. Accept that you are vulnerable and need lots of tender loving care.

Mood scale

5 - Suicidal

4 - Want to run away

3 - Don't want to get up

2 - On verge of tears

1 - Get angry easily

0 - Feel generally miserable

Crying all the time

This is towards the extreme end of the mood swing spectrum and a distressing symptom of the menopause. And it is one, if you are an emotional person, which you are almost certain to encounter. There is probably every indication, if you are crying constantly over nothing or something extremely trivial, that counselling or a hormone replacement –

oestrogen – is called for. If you have a sympathetic doctor, he will understand it is not a case of you just being a weak, weepy woman but that your hormones are seriously playing you up.

Depression

Depression is something much more serious and should not be confused with the feeling of being 'down' which we all get from time to time. Women often say they are 'depressed' when really they mean miserable or fed up: moods which can definitely be traced back to high-low hormonal swings.

Symptoms of real depression are complete lack of concentration, loss of appetite, weight and sex drive, persistent feelings of impending doom, guilt, hopelessness and worthlessness, slow and quiet speech, waking in the early hours, undue fatigue and an inability to take decisions.

If you are clinically depressed you will not be able to perform normal, everyday tasks, keep a diary of everything you do – or don't do – in order to present a coherent picture to your doctor.

Although anti-depressant drugs may be of help to some women, I would suggest a course of therapy first. Professional counselling is becoming more readily available as people, and their doctors, acknowledge that some psychological illnesses can be cured through listening and talking.

Low self-esteem is often at the bottom of depression and this can certainly be made worse by the onset of menopausal problems but there may be other underlying causes which are far more relevant, and good counselling is generally extremely beneficial – HRT may also help.

Headaches

Migraine headaches tend to disappear during the menopause although some women who have never experienced a period headache start to suffer from blinding flashes of pain for the first time. If they are prolonged you should talk it over with your doctor because there could be other causes such as a brain tumour (very rare) or an allergy to certain foods.

The menopause itself does not generally cause headaches although the anxiety associated with it can bring them on. You may come across the term 'vasomotor instability' which means your nerves being affected by hormonal changes. This has a knock-on effect on the walls of blood vessels causing them to dilate and this may result in high blood pressure, so if you are getting frequent headaches which you cannot easily get rid of with aspirin you should get medical advice. There are also some natural headache remedies to try, details of which are later in this book.

Chapter five

Hormonal happiness

Getting the right balance

Hormones get the blame for a lot of things, often with good reason. And you will not be surprised to learn that the word 'hormone' comes from the Greek verb 'to excite'. They are the body's sexual messengers, relaying the needs of the brain or the body to target areas via the blood stream and stimulating organs into action. It is getting the balance right that is so essential to your well being throughout life, but even more so during the menopause.

The hypothalamus is a funnel-shaped central mechanism in the brain which acts as a monitor of all the hormonal activities in the body.

Location of glands in the body

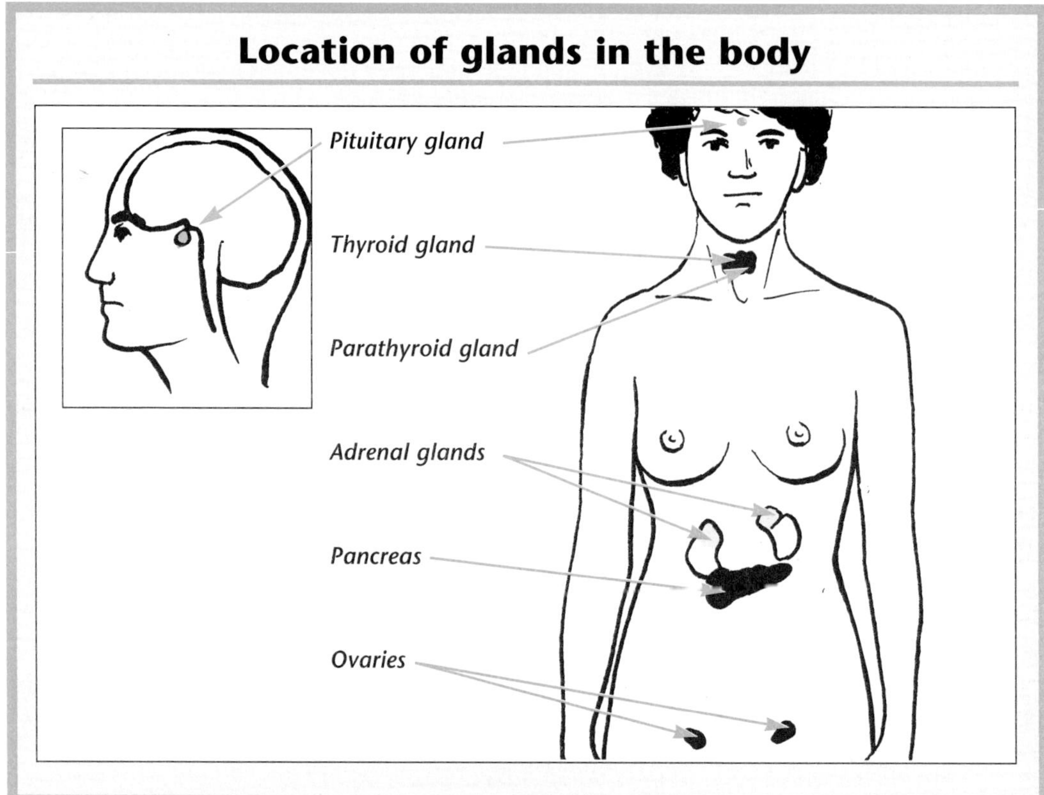

The brain

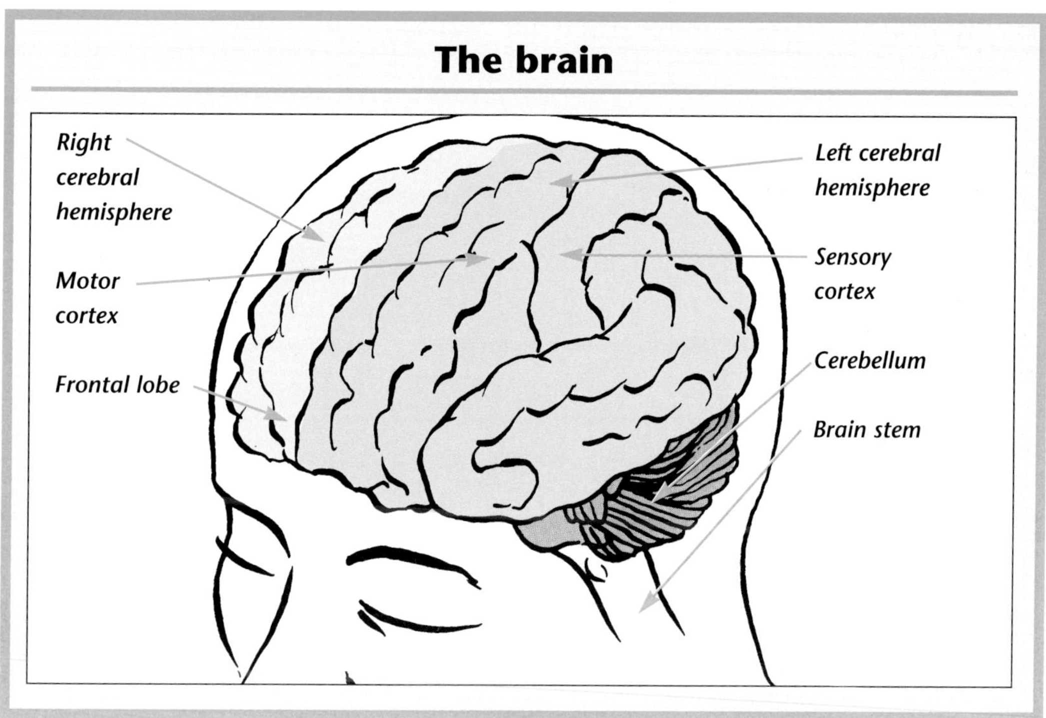

The pituitary is a pea-sized gland at the base of the brain which produces numerous hormones, some influential in the procreative cycle. The first is a follicle stimulating hormone (FSH) and the second, a luteinising hormone (LH). These are the hormones which directly affect the growth and development of the ovarian follicle. The FSH stimulates the follicle to ripen and the LH matures the egg and causes its release.

To a lesser extent the thyroid which lies at the base of the throat, the adrenal gland on top of the kidneys, the ovaries of women and the testes of men also produce hormones. The ovary, the most powerful gland in a woman's body, produces both oestrogen and progesterone which, in different quantities, are deposited in the bloodstream during the monthly cycle. The actual production of oestrogen during the years of the menopause varies considerably from one individual to another. It doesn't stop altogether or abruptly which means some women still experience the same symptoms – swollen or tender breasts, a tendency to retain fluids, emotional vulnerability – which they have always known and not loved.

Hormones can make you hungrier so if you embark on a course of HRT you may start eating too much, and oestrogens can also cause fluid retention both of which are almost certain to make you put on weight. Advice about weight and water retention is later in this book.

Hormonal happiness

Oestrogen

Oestrogen is the female hormone or, more accurately, group of hormones. There are three, the most powerful being oestradiol, then oestrone and finally oestriol. Seventy per cent of the oestrogens circulating in the bloodstream are 'bound' to a specific protein and are finally broken down by the liver.

Oestrogen attaches itself to the surface of cells and plays an important part in much of our general well-being as well as specifically feminine health.

What oestrogen does

- In puberty it causes the enlargement of the breasts.
- Influences pubertal growth of the uterus and fallopian tubes.
- Stimulates growth of the vulva, vagina and uterus.
- Maintains their muscular tone.
- Stimulates secretions of the cervix, particularly at mid-cycle, so creating a favourable environment for male sperm to swim in.
- Helps the endometrium (lining of the womb) to repair and thicken itself following menstruation.
- The muscular capabilities of the tubes are aided by oestrogen.
- Eases the passage of eggs down the fallopian tubes.
- Is involved with the maintenance of the walls of blood vessels.
- Improves blood circulation.
- Is responsible for the formation of the duct system in the breast.
- And the formation of fatty tissue, as well as its pigmentation.
- Offers protection to our bones because it helps to increase the retention of calcium.
- Acts on the blood to decrease cholesterol.
- Maintains the supply of collagen to the skin.
- Affects the condition of our hair.
- Plays an important role in the production of energy.
- Can have a positive effect on our mood, especially during the first two weeks of the menstrual cycle.

Progesterone

Progesterone prepares the womb for the fertilised egg and the mammary glands for milk secretion. After ovulation, the empty follicle (a sac with an egg and fluid in the ovary) collapses in on itself to form a tiny yellowish-red mass of tissue on the surface of the womb. This is called the corpus luteum and it is this substance which produces progesterone. It is also produced by the placenta during pregnancy. Why it is so vital to have enough of it during the menopause is because it protects the lining of the uterus from increasing in thickness by shedding the endometrium.

What progesterone does

- Acts synergistically with other hormones, in particular oestrogens.
- Maintains pregnancy through an intricate hormonal interaction.
- Lessens cervical secretions by changing mucus from a thin and watery substance to one which is thicker.
- Diminishes muscular activity of the uterine wall.
- Contributes to water and salt retention in the body.
- Stimulates growth of milk-secreting cells in the breast tissues.
- Tends to reduce the acidity level of the vagina.
- Raises the base body temperature at the time of ovulation.
- Enhances the immune system through intricate links with prostaglandins and immunoglobulins.
- Influences mood (often for the worse) during the second half of the menstrual cycle.

Androgen

Andogrens are produced by the ovaries long after the menopause and continue to influence our general health and sexuality. They are similar to male hormones and help to maintain muscular strenght and sex drive. Some androgens are converted to oestrogen in the body's fat cells so women with more fat on their bodies produce more oestrogen after the menopause and may have fewer problems with hot flushes, vaginal dryness and brittle bones.

Hormonal happiness

Testosterone

Women do produce some testosterone though obviously far less than men; however, what testosterone women do have may start to have more impact during the menopause. Reduced levels of oestrogen means a woman's body may not be able to counteract the effects of testosterone which can result in facial hair that was not evident before. In rare cases, a menopausal woman's disinterest in sex is due to a lack of free testosterone, and it is well worth seeking expert medical opinion rather than taking it for granted that the problem is psychological.

The male menopause – myth or reality?

There is no such thing as a male menopause. There can't be because men don't have periods. Do they just want to get in on the act because women are getting rather more sympathy today? Do they need an excuse for unacceptable behaviour and even an irrational one will do? I have heard discussions of men whose philandering was attributed to 'the male menopause' when in fact they were philanderers all their lives. This time their wife probably decided enough was enough and booted them out. But some men do have menopausal symptoms like hot flushes, aches and pains, depression and loss of libido, and probably need counselling.

Middle-aged men do sometimes change their staid Volvo for a flashy sports car, leave their wives for a young woman the same age as their daughter and start changing nappies probably for the first time. It can be called 'the male menopause' but it is a misappropriation of the term.

There are some biological changes going on in men but they are very, very gradual. Most don't suffer the chemical chaos raging in our bodies. The testis is to a man what the ovary is to a woman, a gland with two functions: reproduction and hormone production but there is a fundamental difference which is what the menopause is all about. Whereas an ovary is born carrying its eggs and releases them every month, a man's testis can produce spermatozoa throughout his life: there is very little relevant difference between his output at 16 and 60 although not much statistical research has been done. It hardly matters since even a small amount would be enough to do what it is there for.

Testosterone increases in males during puberty and remains constant until they are 45 when it gradually declines. Both sexes have some hormone of the opposite sex circulating in their blood but what is relevant to a man's sex drive is the amount of free testosterone available, which generally decreases with the advancing years. This can sometimes be helped by doctors who specialize in hormone treatment.

How active a man is sexually when he is older very much depends on how active he was when he was younger. This general rule applies to erections which anyway will take longer to develop as a man gets older, but they take much longer or cannot be sustained at all by men who were not very active sexually when they were young. A survey revealed that of men who were the least sexually active earlier, 75 per cent had problems achieving and sustaining an erection in later life; among the moderately active group the figure was 46 per cent and the most active had the least trouble, 19 per cent.

But there are many causes of failing to get an erection. At least 60-70 per cent have an organic cause and should be investigated by a specialist. The more gradual the failure to get an erection, the more likely the cause is physical. If it is sudden, the cause is probably psychological, usually due to anxiety. In older men, erections not only take longer to develop, but may require more direct tactile stimulation; psychic stimulation becomes less and less sufficient. Tactile sensitivity, however, also declines and the period during which an erection can be sustained gets shorter.

Attitudes to sexuality vary across cultures and it seems to be perfectly acceptable in ours for men well into their middle-age to have nubile young women hanging on their arms. The reason, of course, is historical. In former times so many women died in childbirth it was not unnatural to expect a widower to marry again; his new wife would obviously be younger. Luckily for women today, attitudes are changing and it is no longer a matter for raised eyebrows if an older woman has a much younger male partner.

A survey of human relations covering 106 societies worldwide revealed that in twenty-two of them elderly females were sexually active and there was often evidence of lessening sexual inhibitions in older women, leading them to be more openly expressive of their sexual wishes. Sexual relations between old women and much younger men were not considered unusual. Evidently toy boys are neither a modern nor a Hollywood invention.

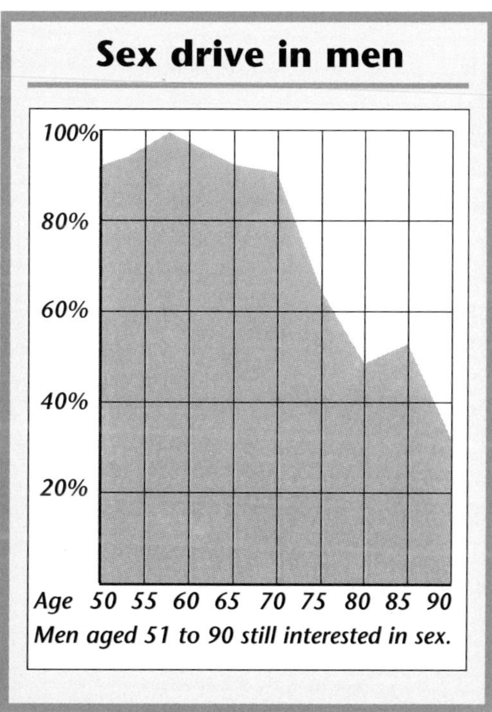

Chapter six

Hormone replacement therapy

Some people claim hormone replacement therapy (HRT) is the best invention since penicillin. Others warn of the dangers inherent in putting chemicals into your system over a long period of time. They argue that the evidence supporting the use of sex hormones is based on too few patients, women who are unrepresentative and that the research is financed by international drug companies with a vested interest in the results. There is also a philosophical argument that women should not be encouraged to try and stave off what is a perfectly natural process – ageing.

Only you can decide on which side of the fence you belong. Much will depend on your own medical history and personal experience of the menopause. If you suffer severe symptoms obviously they will affect your judgement. If you are hardly aware of

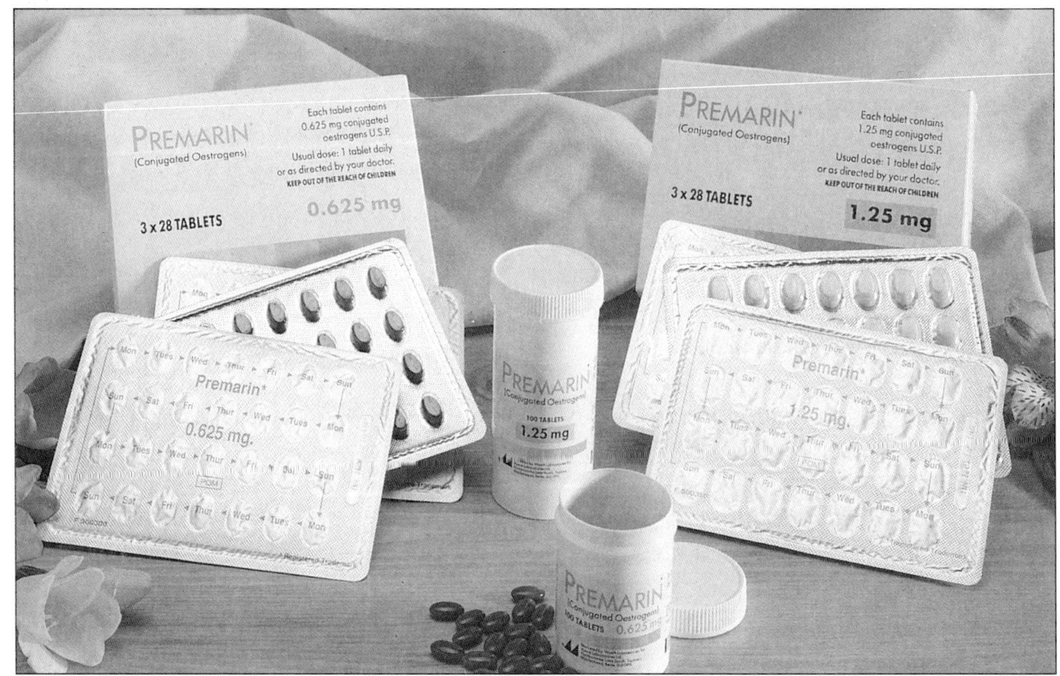

any change the arguments for and against will be more difficult to disentangle. Some of the worries about HRT may not be applicable to you or they may be very relevant. It is a fiercely controversial subject and one about which there are many opposing medical opinions, some of which I will write about in the next chapter. It can be useful to talk to other women to find out what their experience is but in the final analysis only you, with the help of your doctor, can make up your mind. It is your body.

What is hormone replacement therapy?

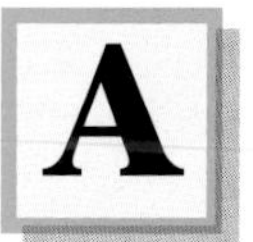

It is literally putting back into your system the hormones your body still needs but is no longer producing enough of for itself. Unlike the contraceptive pill which is used to suppress ovulation, HRT is less potent. You can take either oestrogen on its own (unopposed), a combination of oestrogen and progestogen (opposed), or, rarely, progesterone on its own. The commonest source of most natural oestrogens is extracted from the urine of pregnant mares.

The hormone concentration in your bloodstream bears no relation to the severity or otherwise of menopausal symptoms. What symptoms you get is very much the luck of the draw – and some heredity factors. Although it will be natural to pay more attention to your menopause if it gives you grief, as far as taking a hormone replacement is concerned, many of the benefits are preventative so it is as well to consider the pros and cons of HRT even if you are sailing through the change.

There are a confusing number of hormone replacement preparations, and different ways of taking them, and dosage depends on whether they are natural or synthetic, used in combination or alone and how they affect you personally. Which one suits you best will be dictated by your symptoms, medical history and preference.

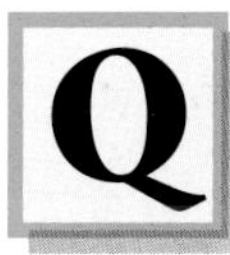

Who takes HRT?

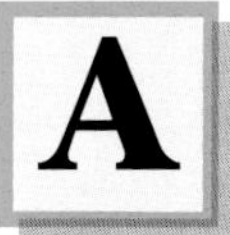

In the UK only 10 per cent of women who are eligible take a hormone replacement, compared to 80 per cent in Canada and the USA. This is probably due to the fact that they receive poor counselling. ERT (oestrogen only) was first used in the 1950s mainly to control hot flushes, vaginal dryness and urinary problems.

Why take it?

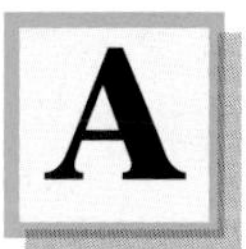

There are several good reasons for taking HRT. Three out of every four women experience menopausal symptoms from the merely uncomfortable to the seriously distressing. Hormone replacements can alleviate many of them, such as:

- Relief from hot flushes and night sweats.

Hormone replacement therapy

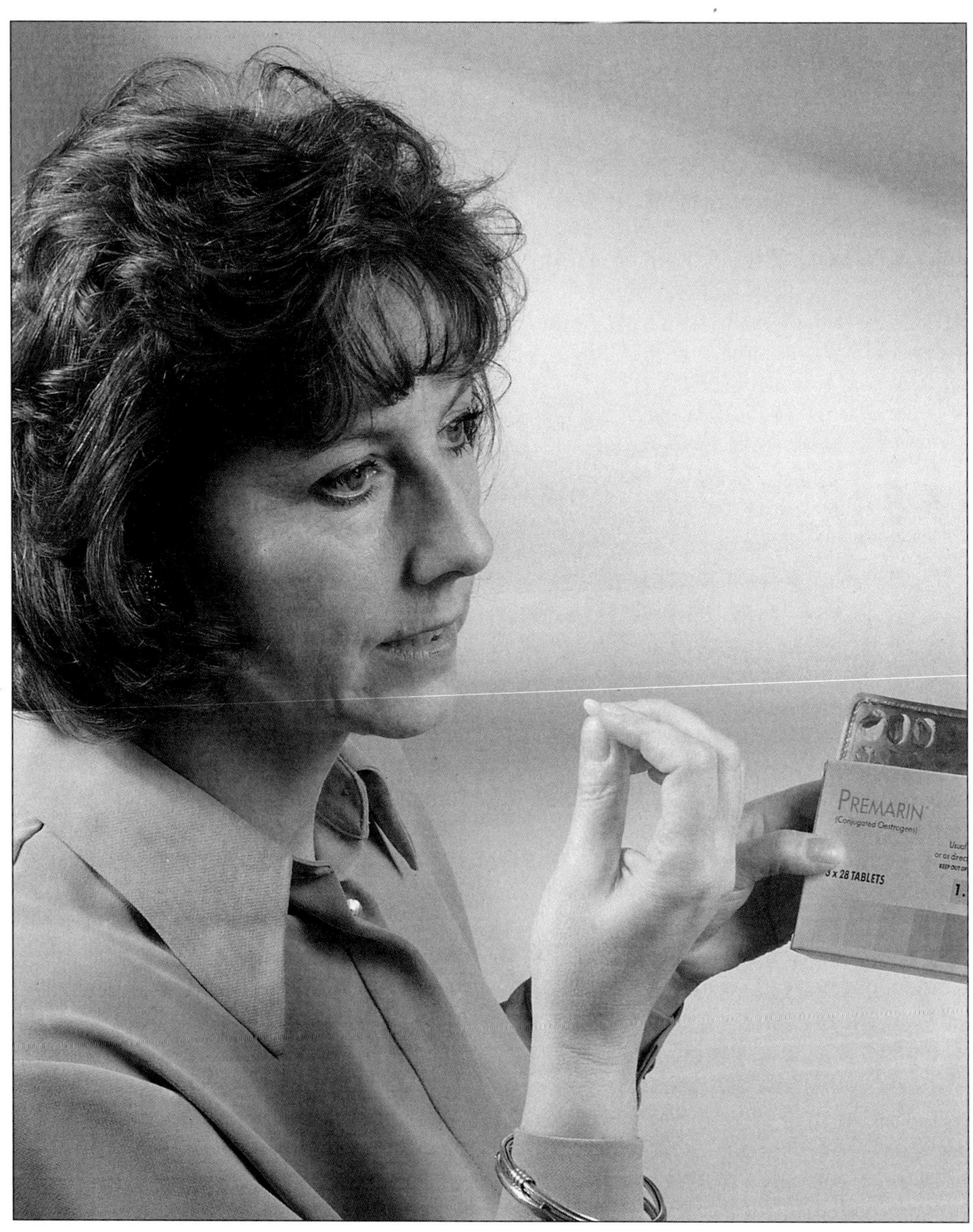

- Prevention of osteoporosis and reduction of risk of fractures.
- Protection against coronary heart disease and stroke.
- Maintenance of skin, keeping it smoother, thicker and softer.
- Benefits to the central nervous system including improvement of memory and sleep.
- Improvement in the lining of the vagina and improvement in vaginal fluids.
- Better bladder control.
- More interest in sex.
- General feeling of well-being.

Who should not take it?

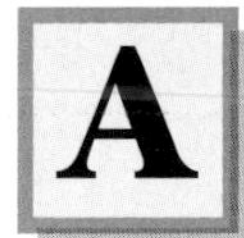

If you have any of the following conditions or there is a family history of these illnesses, you will probably not be prescribed HRT:

- Known or suspected oestrogen-dependent cancers like breast or uterine cancer.
- Abnormal and unexplained genital bleeding (although once it has been investigated, and dealt with, HRT can most likely be prescribed).
- Chronic jaundice or liver disease (although it may be possible to have an HRT patch).
- Undiagnosed lump in breast.
- Present severe thrombosis.

If you suffer from any of the following, careful evaluation ought to be carried out before a course of treatment is prescribed, although normally HRT can be given:

- Uterine fibroids.
- Endometriosis.
- High cholesterol.
- Severe varicose veins.
- Diabetes.
- High blood pressure.
- Thrombosis.
- Liver disease.
- Obesity.
- Gall bladder disease.
- Otosclerosis.

Fibroids

Uterine fibroids are oestrogen-dependent and may increase in size with HRT. Some can grow to be as big as a 16-18 week pregnancy. They can be monitored by pelvic examination and ultrasonography but if they are causing significant problems then usually you have three choices: either stop taking HRT, have a partial hysterectomy or remove the fibroid.

Endometriosis

In endometriosis each case has to be judged on its merits. A laporoscopy would reveal wether it needs treatment and if HRT could be given.

High cholesterol

If you have a high level of cholesterol it will be important which type of hormone replacement you choose. Your doctor will advise you which doses are lipid-friendly.

Severe varicose veins

Severe varicose veins do not rule out HRT provided they are not acutely inflamed (phlebitis). You need to stop taking HRT a month before any leg operation.

Diabetes

Diabetes must be monitored very closely during the first few months of treatment and may require adjustment. Both oestrogens and progestogens effect carbohydrate metabolism though the adverse effects on glucose tolerance are less with HRT combinations than the much more powerful oral contraceptives. Some doctors believe that because people with diabetes are already at increased risk of damage to blood vessels, HRT may not be advisable. But some female diabetics report a tremendous improvement in their quality of life when they take HRT. Obviously it will depend on how disabling your menopausal symptoms are.

High blood pressure

In high blood pressure a non-oral route of administration may be preferable.

Thrombosis

Natural oestrogens do not appear to increase this condition and a non-oral prescription is recommended so the liver is by-passed and fewer metabolic changes are incurred.

Gall bladder disease

Gall bladder disease can be adversely affected by oestrogen due to changes in bile composition and the greater risk of gallstones.

Liver disease

Liver disease may rule out HRT if it is seriously dysfunctional although oestrogen by a non-oral route would avoid compromising the liver further. And if the dysfunction is only temporary there is nothing to stop HRT being prescribed.

Obesity

The arterial risks associated with obesity are not worsened by the administration of HRT although you would have to be carefully monitored.

Otosclerosis

Otosclerosis is an unusual and possibly hereditary condition which produces hardening and fixation of the small bones in the middle ear and, according to some reports, may be made worse with HRT.

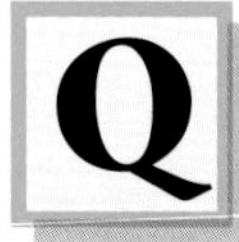

When should you start?

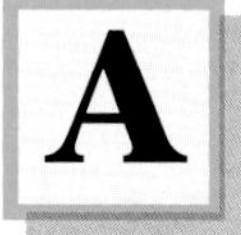

Ideally, during the perimenopausal years, as soon as you start experiencing the first symptoms. The disadvantage, though, is that your hormones will be in a state of flux so it may be difficult to assess exactly what dosage you require. If you only have mild symptoms a small oestrogen supplement during the premenstrual week – if you can still gauge when that is – may be all that is needed.

You can always have a three-month trial period of HRT therapy to see how it suits you. It is highly unlikely you would suffer any serious long-term consequences and it would give you a chance to see if it does or doesn't agree with you. Anything less than three months is unlikely to give you relief from, for instance, hot flushes. The down-side of having a taster is that therapy could provoke, say, irregular bleeding because of the difficulty of getting the hormonal balance right, which could put you off HRT for ever. Counselling from a sympathetic doctor or nurse will allay your worries.

It will be crucial to monitor your response during the trial period. If your troublesome symptom disappears you will know it was due to oestrogen deficiency. Unfortunately, if it doesn't go away, that does not prove the contrary. If only our bodies were that simple. You may have more than one symptom and may need an increased dose. Some women respond better, depending on what disturbances they are encountering, to a hormone replacement administered orally, others when they are administered by other methods. It is important to go back to your doctor so your hormone replacement is tailored to suit you.

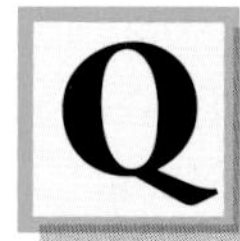

Can women take HRT indefinitely?

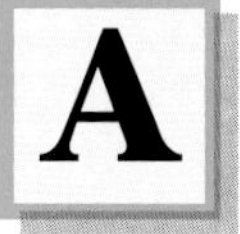

Yes. There is no reason why not if you are satisfied with the treatment. At least two years is recommended for the cessation of most symptoms but there is no reason why women should not continue to take oestrogens into old age.

What types of HRT are there?

Although there are other types of HRT, in practice four are mostly used. You can take them by mouth, as a skin patch, an implant, or vaginal cream.

Oral

At present this is the commonest way of taking oestrogen. The hormone is taken into the bloodstream and then to the liver where it is metabolised. But studies have indicated that anything from 30-90 per cent of the oestrogen taken this way may be inactivated therefore higher doses need to be prescribed to achieve a satisfactory result. As a consequence, occasional nausea is often reported by women who take HRT orally. Oestrogen taken by mouth may also add to the risk of high blood pressure although other factors, especially obesity, play a major role in this. If you are already prone to hypertension you should, perhaps, consider another method.

If you are taking other drugs they might interfere with the absorption rate of an oral oestrogen making it ineffective. And in its passage through the gut, the orally administered oestrogen could also have a negative influence on the production of proteins and anti-blood clotting factors which are carried out principally by the liver.

Patches

These are clear, circular pieces of plastic which you stick onto your bottom or thigh twice a week. The disadvantage of the patch is that it may not have such a favourable effect on blood cholesterol as tablets, or your skin could be allergic to it. An important point in its favour is that it by-passes the gastro-intestinal tract. Some are thinner than others, don't cause so much skin irritation and don't come off so easily when you are swimming. One called Evorel is reported to have caused skin irritation to only six per cent of patients compared to other patches which have a higher incidence.

Vaginal creams

Oestrogen can be applied to a target area and absorbed rapidly. Although principally prescribed for atrophic vaginitis (thinning and inflammation of the vagina), oestrogen creams have the capacity to enter the blood stream. Very low doses, 0.1 mg daily, are capable of producing significant changes in vaginal cytology. There is also a small tablet now on the market which can be inserted into the vagina and is equally effective and suitable for long-term use.

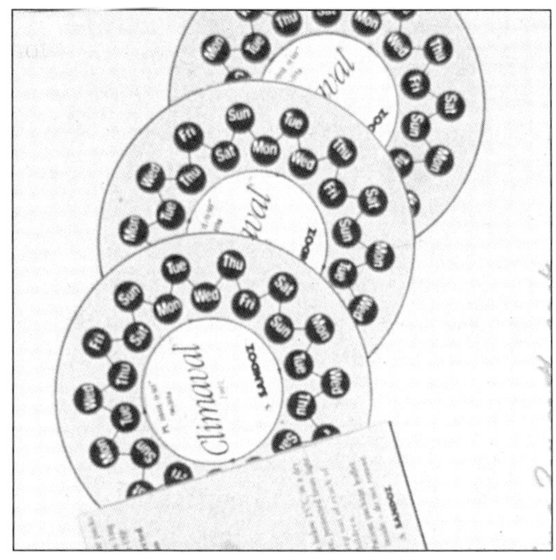

Implants

Subcutaneous oestrogen implants which release their active component over several months have been used for over 30 years but have never really caught on in the UK. They are particularly useful for women who have undergone a hysterectomy as they can avoid taking tablets altogether. An implant has the advantage that you don't have to remember to take it but it is not advisable to take it unless you have had oestrogen therapy before because if it doesn't agree with you, it can be difficult to remove.

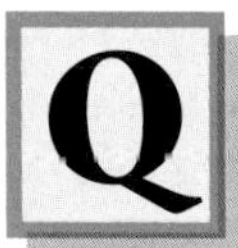

How much HRT should I take?

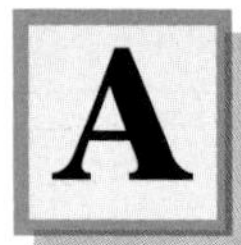

A good rule of thumb is the lowest possible dose except that this will not protect you against bone loss. If you are suffering, or believe that you will be particularly susceptible to osteoporosis, then a higher dose of oestrogen is recommended. It depends which symptoms you are suffering from, how severely and which way of taking HRT you have opted for. Although the ovary produces oestrogen cyclically, for three weeks out of four, it is generally not the pattern followed when taking HRT which is always given continuously – otherwise the troublesome symptoms would surface again every month and the whole point of taking HRT is to rid yourself of those.

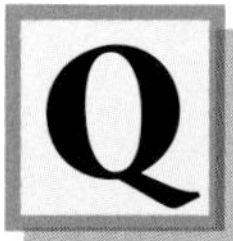

Don't I have to take progestogen as well?

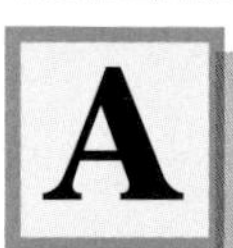

Progestogens (synthetic progesterone) are added to oestrogens to protect the endometrium from cancer. The overwhelming majority of women receive a combined oestrogen-progestogen regimen in which the oestrogen is administered for 28 days and the progestogen is added for 12 days of each monthly cycle Or some doctors recommend 14 days of progestogen every three months.

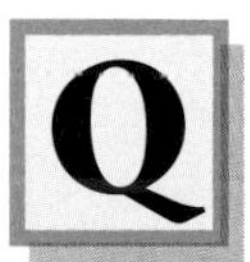

Can I take progestogen on its own?

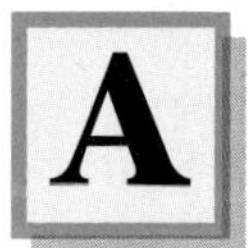

Yes, if you want relief from vasomotor symptoms (hot flushes, night sweats and insomnia) and oestrogen is contra-indicated but then you may increase your risk of heart disease.

Women who were bothered by premenstrual syndrome (PMS) during their reproductive years appear more likely to suffer problems with progestogens postmenopausally.

The effects of progestogen

No large or long-term research has been conducted into the effects of a progestogen-only regime on women going through the menopause but some of the problems connected with this hormone include:

Physical	Psychological
Abdominal cramps	Aggression
Accident-prone	Anxiety
Backache	Apathy
Apathy	Confusion
Breast tenderness	Difficulty making decisions
Dizziness	Forgetfulness
Flatulence	Irrational
General aches and pains	Irritability
Headaches	Panic attack
Hot flushes	Poor concentration
Poor sleep	Tearfulness
Tiredness	
Weight gain	

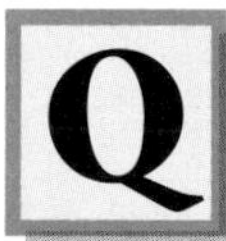

Will I have periods again?

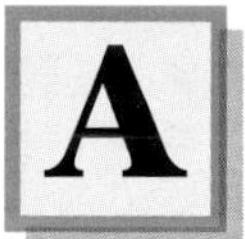

Almost certainly. But it depends whether you take just oestrogen or a combination of oestrogen and progestogen. Eighty five per cent of women who take the combined oestrogen/progestogen regimens experience the re-establishment of withdrawal bleeding. The average woman will bleed for approximately 4-8 days and the flow should resemble that of a normal period experienced during her reproductive phase. However, they usually diminish over time and those women do have peace of mind knowing their endometrium, which could contract cancer, is being sloughed away each month.

Nevertheless it has to be said some women do suffer from heavy bleeding when they take HRT, especially if that is how they menstruated before the menopause and this is a very difficult problem to overcome. Reducing or increasing the oestrogen dose may help but that may also make it less effective. For instance, the protective effect on bone conservation may be lost.

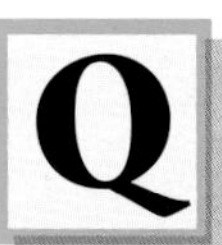

Do hormone replacements cause thrombosis?

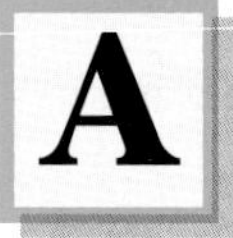

The short answer, according to the Amarant Trust, a charity set up to disseminate information about hormone replacement therapy, is it is very unlikely. Although the production of certain clotting factors may be increased by oral oestrogens, the clinical significance of this is not clear. The answer seems to be that women who are worried they may be at risk of thrombosis should choose a non-oral prescription and have a blood-clotting screen.

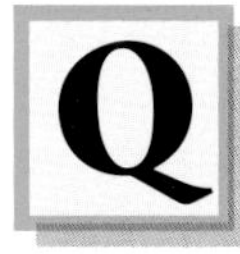

Is there a link between HRT and breast cancer?

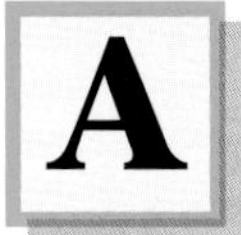

Until recently when it was overtaken by lung cancer, breast cancer was the commonest malignancy in women and the incidence increases with age. One in 12 women in the UK will develop breast cancer during their life. There are many factors which contribute to it. There is evidence that it is related to ovarian cancer and oestrogen status. For example, early age at menarche (when your periods start), obesity (high levels of endogenous oestrogen from peripheral conversion of androgens) and late age of menopause are all associated with an increased risk of breast cancer. Conversely, late menarche and early menopause decrease risk.

Although the risk continues to increase with advancing age, the rate of increase is reduced after menopause and this suggests a lowering of risk associated with reduced oestrogen production. So, will an oestrogen replacement reverse this trend?

There have been a number of worrying press reports claiming breast cancer is not prevented and may even be increased by added progestogens. There is no risk from taking HRT up to five years, and little up to nine years, but thereafter the risk increases although by how much is disputed among doctors.

There is evidence that infertile women whose problem was progesterone deficiency are at greater risk postmenopausally of carcinoma of the breast. If the possibility of getting breast cancer is a serious concern to you – and there is still a great deal of research into the long-term effects of HRT going on – it is worth making yourself aware of all the available medical opinion until you are confident about taking HRT.

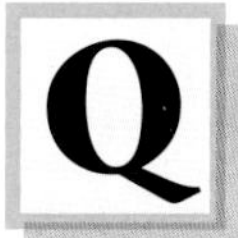

Does HRT affect blood pressure?

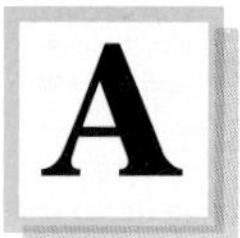

Because the original high-dosage oral contraceptives were associated with transient hypertension in some young women, oestrogen replacement therapy was expected to have a similar effect. The pro-HRT lobby say numerous studies have indicated that most hypertensive patients require less medication after hormone replacement therapy. However, others point out that some widely used progestogens have adverse effects on lipoprotein levels and may raise blood pressure.

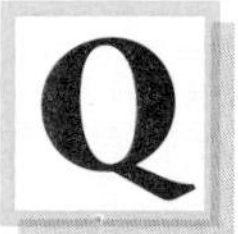

Can I take HRT if I have had a hysterectomy?

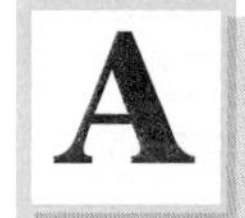

Yes. If you have had a hysterectomy you need only take oestrogen. The combined oestrogen progestogen therapy is prescribed principally to protect the lining of the womb from endometriosis.

Is HRT good for the heart?

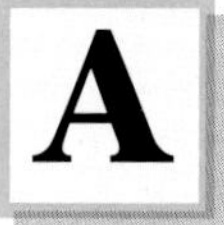

This is probably the most important issue as far as women in general are concerned because arterial disease is the commonest cause of death in women aged over 50 years. It kills approximately one woman in four every year so any benefit from HRT is likely to be a statistically significant one. According to Malcolm Whitehead, a senior lecturer and consultant gynaecologist at King's College School of Medicine, London, "It is now clear that the major public health benefit of oestrogen replacement therapy (ERT) is a reduction of at least 50 per cent in the incidence of coronary heart disease."

It appears that ovarian failure is followed by an increase in total cholesterol and that an oestrogen replacement can have a beneficial influence by increasing the high density lipoprotein (HDL) level compared to the low density lipoprotein (LDL), the 'baddie' as far as a healthy heart is concerned.

What effect does HRT have on osteoporosis?

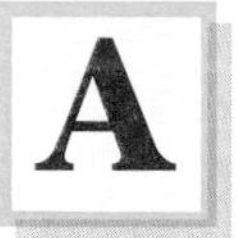

Oestrogens have a role in the prevention of osteoporosis and they may also be beneficial in treating established disease. They help to conserve bone mass and therefore reduce the incidence of fractures of the wrist, spine and hip. As a general rule, the earlier you start taking oestrogens the better because although you can arrest bone loss years after your menopause has started, you can't put back what you have already lost, although you can improve bone density. The minimum time you should take HRT in order to give your bones maximum benefit is three years although women experiencing a premature menopause should take it for at least five. It is not known whether extending the duration of HRT for, say, 10 years will exert greater protective effects. But it has been shown that bone loss resumes after oestrogen withdrawal.

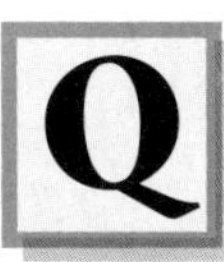

Can HRT help if you suffer from bowel disease?

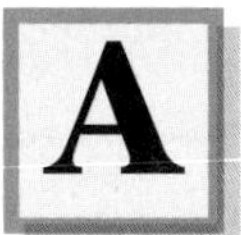

Women with Crohn's disease or ulcerative colitis tend to have an earlier menopause. The damage caused to the gut and the steroid treatment which they receive for their bowel conditions predisposes them to bone loss and osteoporosis. Treatment with HRT prevents further bone loss and increases bone density.

Will HRT stop me from getting old?

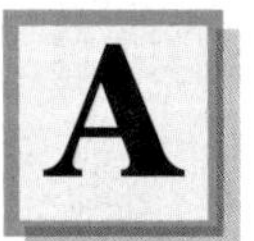

The short answer to that has to be No, although it does put back collagen. But there are signs that it can stave off some ageing diseases. For instance, new American research claims that women who receive oestrogen replacement therapy are less likely to develop Alzheimer's, the leading cause of dementia in the elderly which affects one third of people over the age of 85 robbing them of their memory, understanding and mental processes. Alzheimer's disease is three times more common among women.

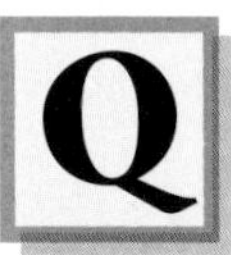

What should I ask my doctor?

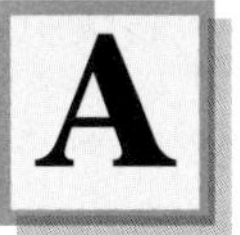

It would be useful to go along for your first consultation with a list of questions. They will depend on your own medical history because any illnesses you have had before, say endometriosis, or deaths your family has suffered, stroke or breast cancer, say, will affect both your judgements. Don't be shy of taking notes of what he is telling you; that's a sensible thing to do because there are a bewildering number of benefit/risk ratios to take into account.

If you decide to go ahead with HRT, ask your doctor how many of the following tests he thinks you may need.

Test check list: Ideally, some of these tests ought to be done every six months, others annually and some only if you think you are susceptible or want to be cautious.

- Blood oestrogen levels.
- Calcium level.
- Bone density.
- Mammogram.
- Blood pressure.
- Cervical cancer smear.

Chapter seven

Food for thought

You are not going to be able to eat your way out of the menopause but your diet plays a crucial role in the way growing older affects you. Scientists now believe that beta-carotene not only helps to protect the skin wrinkling, but it may be especially successful in helping to prevent cancer from occurring. And Professor Khaw who argues against the

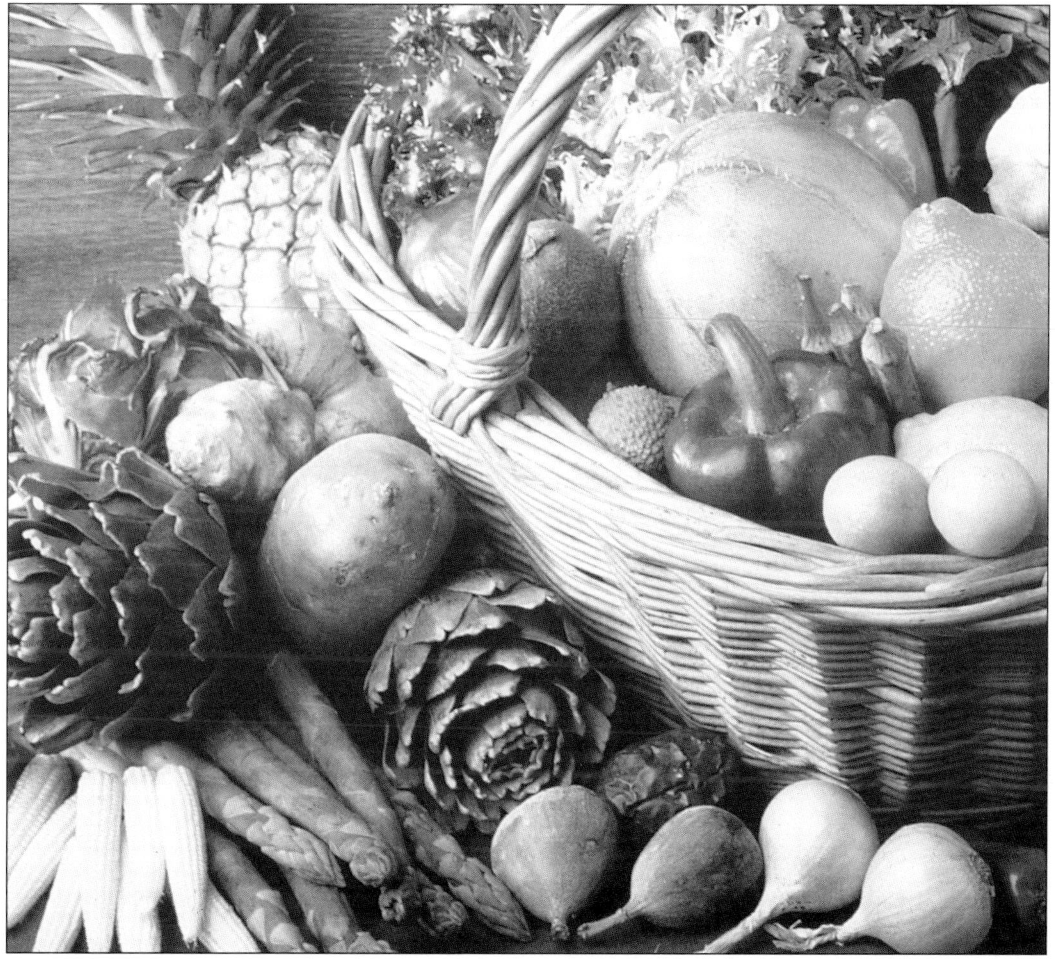

efficacy of oestrogen replacements, points out that natural oestrogens found in many plant foods like beans and pulses could lower the risk of osteoporosis, breast cancer and heart disease. It is never too late to learn healthy eating habits and you will probably find it easier to be disciplined now. There is nothing like coming face to face with a reality like the menopause for concentrating the mind.

Lesson one:

Your metabolism slows down as you get older so your body can tolerate fewer calories. The energy level for women aged 51-75 is estimated at 1800 calories with a range of 1400-2200 compared to 2000 calories with a range of 1600-2400 for women aged 23-50. A 51-year-old woman would have to reduce her daily intake to 1300 calories per day to lose one pound per week. Equally, a very low calorie diet, below 1000 calories, is unlikely to give you the required amount of essential nutrients.

Lesson two:

Work out your body mass index (see below). It is a fairly reliable guide to how healthy you are. The acceptable range for women is between 20-25. If you are under 20 you should have a check up because the menopause could be causing you to lose weight and you may need dietary advice from your doctor. A reading of 20-25 is about average. If you score between 25-30 you should start to pay more attention to what you eat. Between 30-40 and you are beginning to be obese and if you score more than 40 you are seriously unhealthy and should seek medical help immediately.

Your body mass index

To work out your body mass index (BMI) use the following simple equation:

Body mass index = weight in kilograms divided by height in metres squared.

Therefore if you weigh 57kg (9 stone) and are 1.65m (5ft 5in) tall, your body mass index would be 21, which falls within the acceptable range for women of between 20 and 25, and is normal and healthy.

This is a more accurate way of assessing the right weight range for an individual than the old system of height-weight charts. However, nowadays most charts are based on BMI values and ranges.

If you are overweight and want to get slimmer, then talk to your doctor or consider joining one of the weight loss organisations which run weekly classes to help you. Many people benefit from this approach and the encouragement and moral support they receive. Alternatively, you may wish to embark on a more healthy eating plan and an exercise programme.

Lesson three:

Beta-carotene is found in brightly coloured fruit and vegetables (see box below) so make sure you eat plenty every day.

Lesson four:

So long as you are not too overweight, a little bit of fat helps to protect you from osteoporosis because it encourages the production of a type of oestrogen.

Lesson five:

Readjust your priorities. Put raw vegetables at the top of your shopping list; substitute pasta, rice and pulses for meat. Keep the water you cook carrots in (or any other

Beta-carotene

Beta-carotene is measured in micrograms (mcg) and it is estimated we should be aiming for 15,000 a day.
Vegetables should be cooked in a little butter or brushed with olive oil because beta-carotene is fat-soluble.

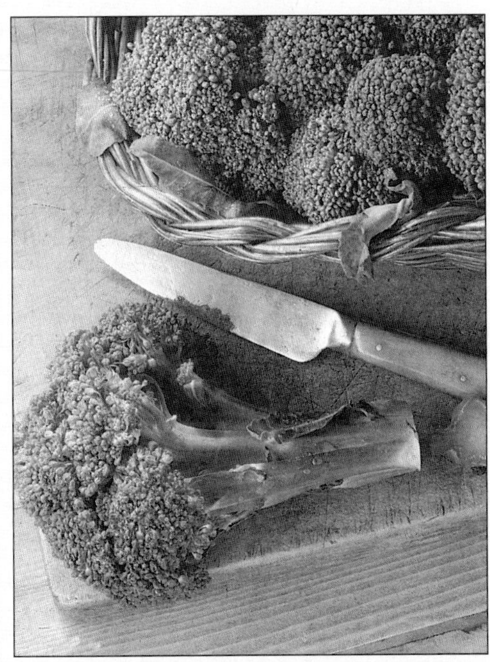

	mcg per 100
Carrots	4425
Parsley	4040
Sweet potatoes	3960
Spinach	3840
Watercress	2520
Spring greens	2270
Cantaloupe melon	1000
Tomatoes	640
Asparagus	530
Broccoli	475
Apricots	405
Peaches	58

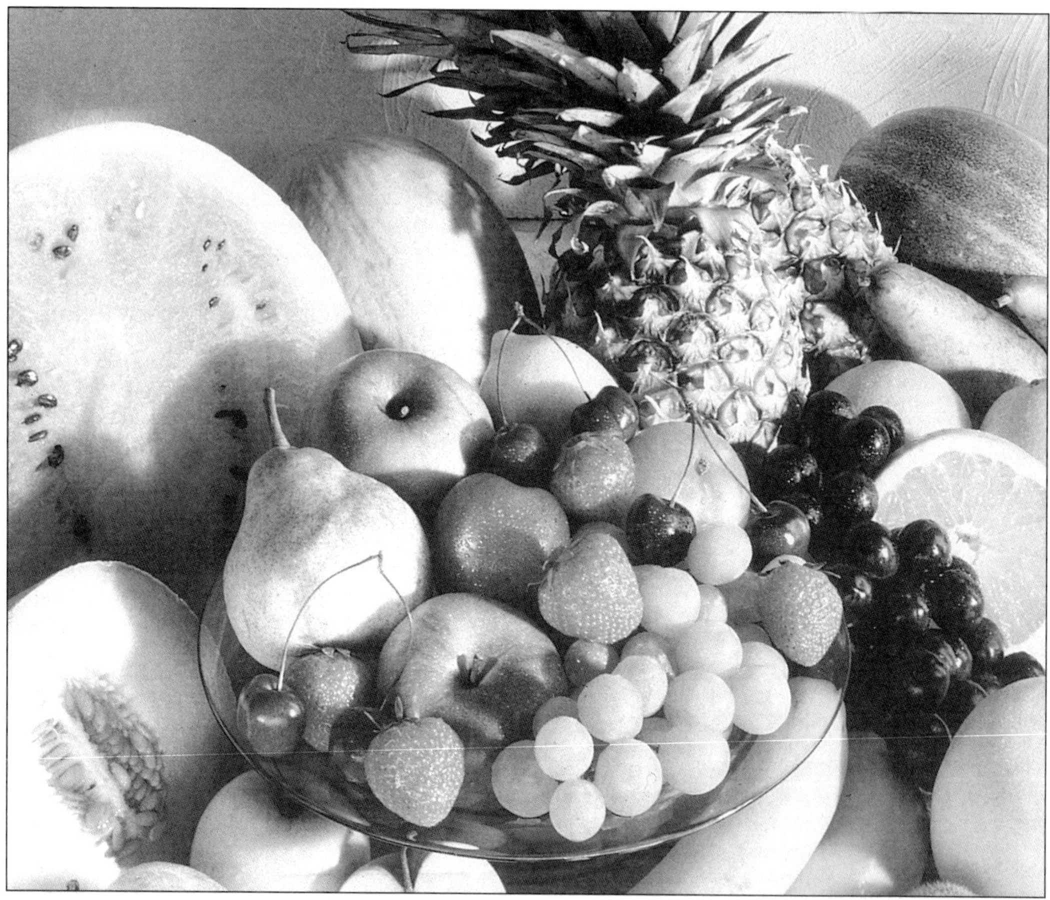

vegetable) because vitamins, especially vitamin C, leech into the water. Why throw it down the drain? Put it into a soup.

Lesson six:

Watch the sugar. It is worrying how much refined sugar we eat – one estimate puts it at 200 lbs a year per head of population in the UK. Sugar has no nutritional value. Once you have made up your mind to give it up you will be surprised at how – relatively – easy it is. Don't attempt to wean yourself off it all at once. Give yourself a year and have a planned programme. Start with one sugar-free gesture and follow up with others such as:

- Cut by half the amount you put in tea/coffee.
- Add banana/apple/pear to unsugared cereal.
- Substitute fizzy drinks for fresh fruit ones.
- Treat yourself to dates/apricots/figs instead of chocolate.
- Experiment with herb teas.

During the menopause you have enough to do coping with mood swings induced by your changing hormones and, often, with a lifestyle that is changing at the same time, without adding to your body's difficulties by flooding your system with sugar. It sets up a chain reaction causing normal blood sugar levels to rise dramatically which overload the pancreas. Often the pancreas can't cope; it has great trouble trying to get the balance right which is why so many women experience extreme fluctuations in mood. High concentrations of glucose in the blood can produce surges of energy and high spirits but these can change just as quickly to feelings of listlessness, hunger and lassitude as the blood sugar level drops.

Lesson seven:

Menopausal women require the same amount of protein, vitamins and minerals as they did when they were young, so there is less room in the diet for high-calorie, low-nutrient foods.

Lesson eight:

Drink as much water as you can: two litres – preferably still water rather than sparkling. You don't want to introduce extra gas into your stomach. However, too much, say 4 litres, can also cause problems.

Lesson nine:

Many women experiencing the menopause also begin to experience constipation. This is partly due to the effects of oestrogen withdrawal and the resultant change in the physiology of the digestive system. Called the 'father of diseases' it can really only be tackled successfully through diet. Make sure you eat enough fibre, drink hot orange juice first thing in the morning or make a mild emetic with grated fresh ginger soaked in hot water. It may also be necessary to increase your vitamin B intake through one or two supplements before each meal.

Note

If you are suffering from unusual mood swings, check first on your sugar intake because it may not be your hormones that are sending you into orbit.

Lesson ten:

Change the habits of a lifetime and stop eating three meals a day. Instead eat five or six but smaller ones. An apple can count as a meal and it is much better to eat it on an empty stomach. Eating this way is better for your digestion which will not be as robust as it once was.

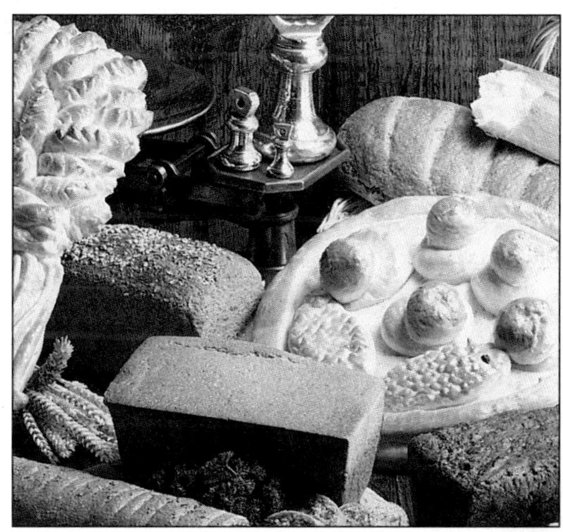

Food for thought

Nutrition

It is impossible to over-emphasise the need for proper nutrition during the menopause. It is always important but while your body is adjusting to so many chemical changes it is crucial you do not starve it of the essential nutrients it needs to function at its best. The Japanese taste for high protein soya-bean products such as tofu may play an important role in the much lower incidence of heart disease, breast cancer and osteoporosis in that country.

Your daily food guide

Fruits and vegetables
Four servings to include one citrus fruit, one dark green or deep yellow fruit or vegetable and two others.

Grains and cereals
Four servings (one slice of bread equals a serving), preferably whole grain.

Protein foods
Two servings: three ounces meat, fish or poultry; one ounce hard cheese, three ounces cottage cheese.

Fats, sweets and alcohol
None – they should be eaten only after the food from the other four groups has been chosen and you should probably not be eating more than 1500 calories a day.

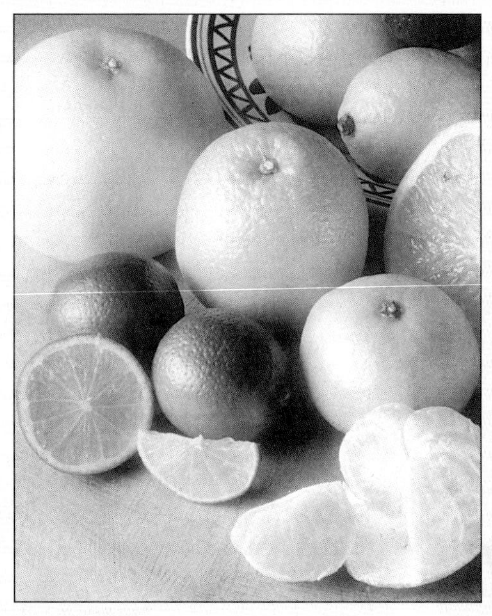

Calcium

The mineral content of bone is mainly calcium and for the menopausal woman it is one of the most important nutrients because changes in the body's calcium metabolism cause bone loss leading to osteoporosis. Calcium deficiency can also contribute to bad nerves and insomnia. Calcium is often called the 'wonder vitamin' because it performs so many functions in the maintenance of good health, including normal blood coagulation, and heart and muscle action. According to the government's latest nutritional advice, women need at least 700 milligrams per day.

As you get older the body absorbs calcium less efficiently and therefore higher levels of dietary calcium are required. This applies particularly for the over-sixties and beyond. Most research indicates that eating more calcium or taking a calcium supplement does not, however, afford the same protection to bones as oestrogen.

Recognising that high calcium intake cannot prevent bone loss due to oestrogen

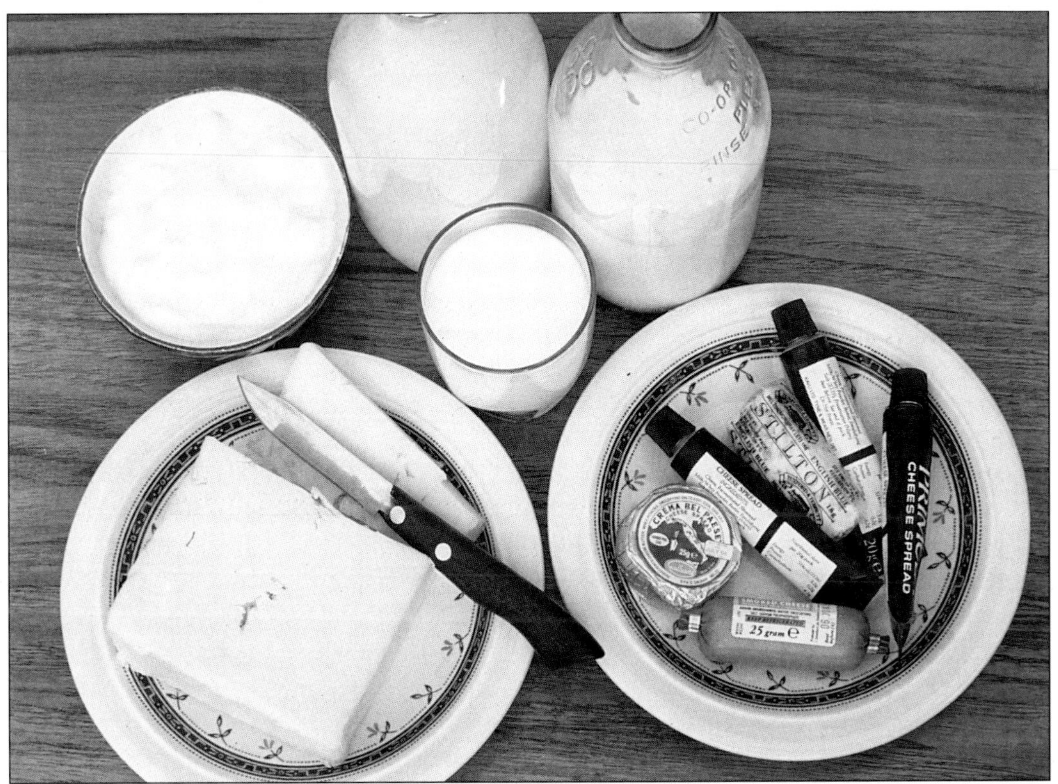

Food for thought

Calcium-rich foods

1 pint milk: whole, low-fat or skimmed	670mg
Cheddar cheese 100g	380mg
Cottage cheese 100g	60mg
Canned sardines (or salmon) 100g	550mg
Milk chocolate 100g	200mg
Yogurt	400mg

Other foods containing calcium

- Broccoli.
- Soya flour.
- Kale.
- Dates.
- Cabbage.
- Beans.
- Cauliflower.
- Dried fruit.
- Turnip.
- Molasses.
- Meat and bacon.
- Almond and Brazil nuts.
- Wheatgerm.
- Tofu.
- White bread.

deficiency, it is still prudent to avoid adding the additional insult of calcium deprivation.

Because menopausal women are often worried about putting on weight they are sometimes reluctant to increase the amount of calcium-rich foods they eat. Women also fear dairy products will cause constipation and some have lactose intolerance, so if you fall into one of those categories, a calcium supplement may be a necessity. However, it is important to remember that low-fat dairy products contain as much calcium as full-fat varieties.

Calcium cannot be absorbed without vitamin D and is also affected by certain drugs such as antacid medicines and the corticosteroids, if they are used for long periods. Since vitamin D is obtained from sunlight and can be absorbed through the skin most of us get plenty during the spring and summer but in the autumn and winter it is important to make sure your diet contains some vitamin D. Alcohol directly prevents absorption of calcium and so do bran, wholewheat pasta and large amounts of wholemeal bread, which contains a substance called phytic acid. This also blocks the absorption of magnesium, iron, zinc, copper and vitamin B. So although you need some fibre in your diet, especially if you tend to get constipated, it is better to get it from legumes, fruit, vegetables and salad. (White bread is fortified with calcium, iron and some B vitamins.)

Although calcium is present in spinach and rhubarb, because of other components in those foods, your body cannot absorb the calcium contained in them. Excessive salt intake will also restrict your ability to benefit from calcium in food although a diet high in vegetables and fruit contains a lot of potassium which may counteract the effect of sodium. You can reduce your sodium

Low-fat sources of calcium

Milk, yogurt and cheese are the major sources of calcium in our diet, and, in addition to supplying calcium, they also provide other valuable nutrients like protein, B vitamins and minerals. Many women worry about eating too many dairy products as whole milk and many cheeses are high in fat, and thus calories! However, you can opt for semi-skimmed or skimmed milk, which have all the calcium of whole milk but are lower in fat and calories. For example, a typical 300ml/$^1/_2$ pint glass of whole milk would provide 345mg calcium, whereas the same amount of skimmed milk has 360mg calcium.

Unfortunately, low-fat cottage cheese does not contain as much calcium as a hard cheese, such as Cheddar. Whereas 50g/2oz Cheddar supplies 360mg calcium, you will only get 73mg from eating 100g/3 $^1/_2$oz cottage cheese. However, a small 150g/5oz carton of plain yogurt yields 285mg calcium.

So even if you are on a calorie-controlled slimming diet, you can still ensure that you get adequate amounts of calcium every day without ruining your chances of slimming success. We all know that most of us eat too much fat so it is a good idea anyway to switch to low-fat alternatives.

intake by taking the following steps:

- Don't add salt to food.
- Don't eat fast food as it usually has a high sodium content.
- Avoid anything containing sodium bicarbonate.
- Wash frozen, canned and smoked seafood in cold water.
- Read food labels carefully for added salt.
- Avoid monosodium glutamate, sodium sulphate, sodium chloride and sodium nitrate which are present in many foods.

Heart disease

As I have already said, the incidence of heart attacks among women increases considerably after the menopause – another pressing reason for looking closely at your eating-exercise lifestyle. Check your cholesterol and if it is too high – over 6.5 – give yourself six months to reduce it by switching to fat-free foods.

- Be ruthless and cut down drastically on saturated fats.
- Forget hard cheese exists, except for flavour.
- Cut out any foods with added sugar.
- Reduce the amount of salt you use.
- Never fry anything; instead 'stir-fry' in a thimbleful of oil.
- Introduce lots of pulses into your diet.
- Are you drinking too much alcohol?
- Cut down on your caffeine intake.

Food for thought

Caffeine

Recent research shows that drinking large amounts of caffeine during pregnancy may cause birth defects and many doctors are now advising middle-aged women to look carefully at the amount of caffeine they consume. We know caffeine has a quite profound effect on the nervous system. It stimulates the heart, making it beat more rapidly, and the brain, making you think more quickly. It also temporarily banishes fatigue but, because it causes more acid secretion in the stomach, it can have a detrimental effect on ulcers. With your hormones already in a state of chemical chaos, it makes no sense at all to add to the maelstrom by swallowing litres of what you could describe as straight stress. Caffeine can cause constant feelings of tension and hypersensitivity which can cause disturbances in the output of hormones and even menstrual irregularities.

General sense of well-being

Zinc is well known for its role in growth and tissue repair and is essential for the immune system. It is also involved in hundreds of metabolic pathways maintaining our senses of taste and smell. Other pathways which zinc clears deal with the digestion of carbohydrates and the balance of insulin controlling blood-sugar levels. It helps the absorption of other nutrients, such as vitamin A and the B-complex vitamins, and is one of our most important antioxidants which protect cells.

Soil deficiencies of zinc have reduced the levels available in plant foods and zinc is also removed by food processing. High levels of calcium and phytates found in plant foods are thought to block absorption of zinc from [illegible] The body's stores of zinc can be [illegible] missing meals or fasting. [illegible] g a multi-vitamin, mineral [illegible] day.

Hot flushes

There may be no scientific evidence to prove why, but many women say their hot flushes are relieved by eliminating caffeine, sugar and alcohol from their diets

Water retention

This is a problem for some women throughout their adult life and is exacerbated during the menopause. The biggest culprit is salt and on average we eat about 13 grams ($2\frac{1}{2}$ teaspoonfuls) a day but we only need about three grams (half a teaspoonful). Besides causing loss of calcium it can also lead to high blood pressure which, in turn, can cause heart disease, kidney disease and strokes. Two-thirds of the salt we eat has been added by food manufacturers so:

- Don't add any more, try lemon juice, spices and herbs instead.

Good sources of zinc

- Shellfish.
- Herrings.
- Meat

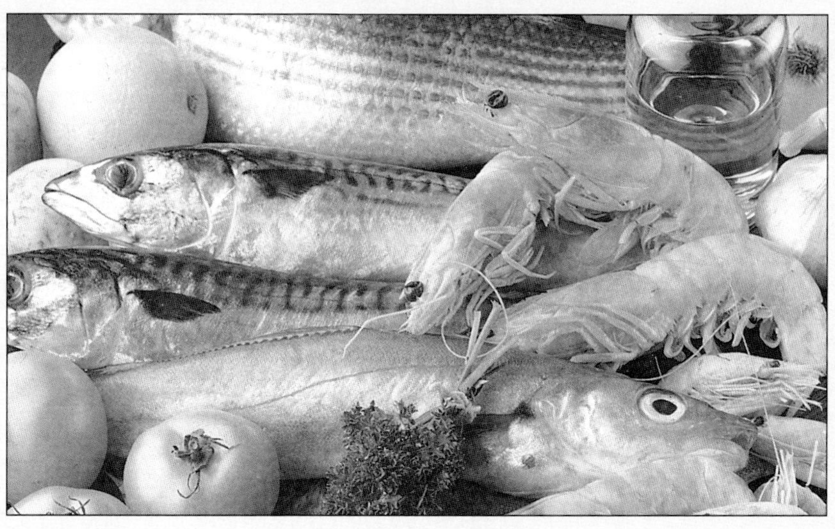

- Stock cubes are very salty.
- So is soya sauce.
- So are packet soups.

Also, eat more natural diuretics such as celery, parsley or grapes and take more exercise because you lose salt in your sweat. Sassafras is a tonic combating fatigue and nervous depression and is beneficial when used after strenuous exercise. It also possesses a diuretic. Make a massage oil by adding 2-4 drops to teaspoons of oil or add the same amount to a warm (not hot) bath.

Whatever you do, don't 'go on a diet'. That is guaranteed to make you fed up. Regard the menopause as a new beginning. The new you has to adopt a completely different pattern of eating: one that is healthy and interesting.

Chapter eight

Get fit for the rest of your life

The highest prevalence of obesity among women is in the 45 to 54 years age group. Middle-aged women often find, to their dismay, they tend to gain weight more easily and have to work harder to lose it than they once did. Although eating habits are generally blamed, it is a fact that resting energy needs diminish by about two per cent per decade throughout adulthood. If not compensated for, this fairly small decline can lead to a substantial weight gain over three decades.

Why exercise?

Taking regular and vigorous exercise is just as important as eating healthily. In an hour of brisk walking, a 60-kilogram woman will use up 200 calories, that is as well as doing her heart a lot of good and helping to maintain her bone mass. If you are stronger and more agile because you exercise, you are less likely to fall over and break bones. Active older people have better coordination, balance and muscular strength than their sedentary peers. Exercise also improves your sense of well-being. In an elevated mood, you are less likely to succumb to tranquillisers or anti-depressants which can lessen your co-ordination.

To avoid brittle bones

For exercise to be osteogenic it needs to be vigorous and diverse. Running, weight training, stair climbing, field sports such as hockey, court games like tennis or squash, and dancing are all recommended. Ideally, these should be undertaken at least four days a week for a minimum of 30 minutes.

Research conducted at the University of Nottingham indicated that a modest amount of jumping, performed daily over a year, increased the density of hip bones in premenopausal women by a substantial three per cent. The women performed only 50 jumps a day which takes less time than cleaning your teeth.

Weight-bearing physical activity is essential for bone health. When mechanical stress or gravitational force on the skeleton is removed, if you are bedridden, for instance, bone loss is rapid and extensive. Professional athletes, on the other hand, usually have above-average bone mass.

By far the most effective exercise programme is one which you will keep to.

A sensible option, if avoiding the onset of osteoporosis is a major concern, would be to join a gym where you can learn how to use weights. There will be a trained instructor who will be able to control your work-out programme so that, over a period of time, you can gradually increase your bone strength.

To help your heart

Aerobic activities such as running, swimming or cycling are all good exercises to achieve cardiovascular fitness, but they have to be undertaken fairly vigorously and on a regular basis. The object of the exercise must be to get your blood pumping faster round your body, raising your heart beat and your oxygen intake.

To lower cholesterol

It generally takes four months of vigorous exercise, like walking on a motorised treadmill for 30 minutes three times a week, to have any impact on high-density lipoprotein levels. Other fairly strenuous activities, such as running between 10-15 miles a week or walking 30 miles, will give the same benefit.

To improve your sex life

Wherever you are, standing at a bus stop, waiting for a train, watching the kettle boil or lying in bed, you can do the following famous exercise.

Imagine you want to stop urinating by firmly squeezing the muscles in your vaginal area. Slowly count to three then relax. Repeat this squeeze-and-hold at least ten times a session and remember to do it three or four times a day. The exercise was invented by a gyneocologist to help women overcome vaginal atrophy which often results in the distressing passing of water when you sneeze or cough. It strengthens the muscles and teaches you how to control them.

To make you feel good

The secretion of a number of hormones, particularly those of the gonads and pituitary, are influenced by exercise. Insulin sensitivity increases, as shown by the body's ability to take up and utilise glucose in response to a smaller amount of insulin, and its release from the pancreas decreases.

Some studies have shown that aerobic exercise performed for 12 weeks reduced depression (in patients complaining of mild to moderate depression) to a greater degree than traditional psychotherapy. They were also still in a depression-free state when evaluated 12 months later. Peripheral levels of endorphins rise with exercise but less is known about whether this is responsible for the 'feel good' factor most people report after exercising. A sense of well-being and achievement as well as a feeling of relaxation are bonuses to the health benefits regular exercise offers.

To stop that feeling of fatigue

Ageing decreases the body's capacity for energy generation in muscle. The metabolism of glucose and free fatty acids, essential for muscle strength, is greatly assisted by exercise, therefore the physically inactive older woman puts herself even more at risk of tiredness by not assisting her body to regenerate its own energy stores. Rhythmic exercise results in the exercised muscle becoming more resistant to fatigue.

To stop your joints seizing up

Whether it happens just before, during, or soon after the menopause, one of the more horrible signs of getting older is that stiffness as you rise from your cinema seat or armchair. Besides eating plenty of oily fish which you should have been doing all your life, the only other way to overcome joint stiffness is by exercising regularly.

Regular activity maintains the nutrition of articular cartilage while inactivity or immobilisation results in atrophy. The stability of a joint depends upon the supporting ligaments and the surrounding muscles, and the balance between the different muscle groups acting on a joint is responsible for maintaining the dynamic stability of that joint. Swimming for at least half an hour two or three times a week, doing a variety of strokes, will help to keep the joints mobile.

What you can do to keep the joints jumping

- It is important to do stretching exercises as soon as you get up in the morning and before you take off on any vigorous exercise programme.
- Reach above your head as far as you can stretch, hands clasped together. Hold for a count of ten. Feel the muscles in your shoulders and arms being stretched.
- Reach your hands behind your back and clasp them together for a count of ten. The muscles in your shoulders and upper back will be loosened and strengthened by this exercise.
- Bend to the side from the waist, stretching your opposite hand over your head. Start with three and work up to as many as you can manage. You will feel muscles down the side of your back and your waist being stretched.
- Twist from the waist to face the wall behind you, keeping your hips straight and stomach in. Feel the effect in your lower back, tummy and waist.
- Sit on the floor and place the soles of your feet together. Holding your toes, bring your feet as close to your body as you can, pushing your knees towards the floor. This stretches the inside thigh muscles.
- Stand on one leg, bend the other leg behind you and hold your foot to a count of 10, the front of your thigh muscle being pulled. Repeat with the other leg.

Your posture

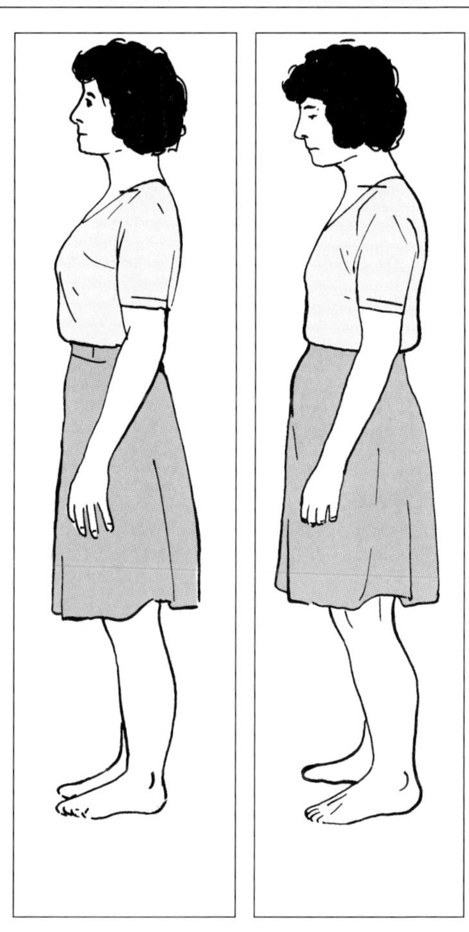

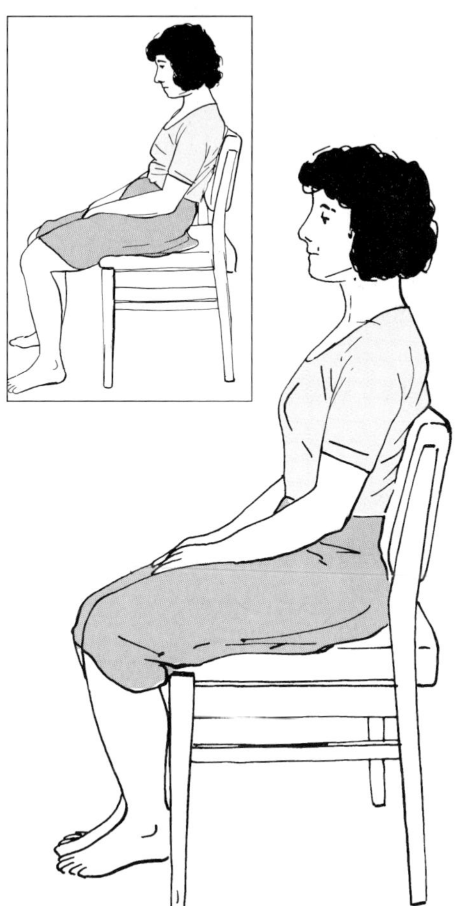

Good posture is important. Try not to 'slump' with hunched shoulders and stomach sticking out; this puts pressure on your spine. Stand up straight and walk tall with shoulders back and stomach pulled in. Your weight should be evenly distributed between both legs. Sit up straight in a comfortable chair which supports your lower back; don't slouch.

Breathing exercises

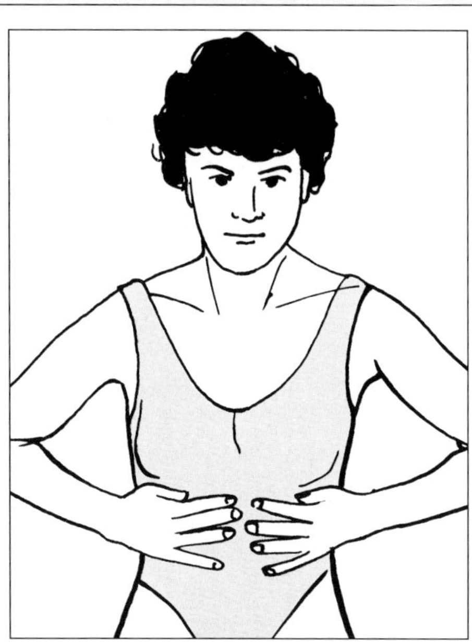

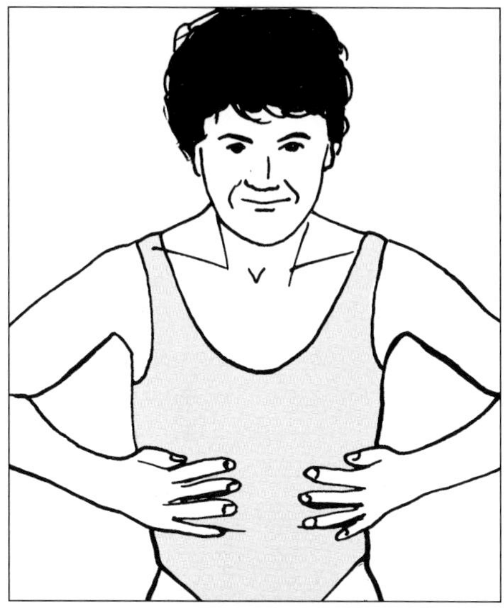

These will help retain elasticity and mobility in the rib cage and prevent you becoming short of breath. Above: with hands on either side of your rib cage, breathe in deeply. Feel your hands moving outwards and upwards with the ribs. Repeat 3 times. Right: clench a fist tightly and place it in the gap between the ribs. Inhale and feel your tummy rising. Repeat 3 times.

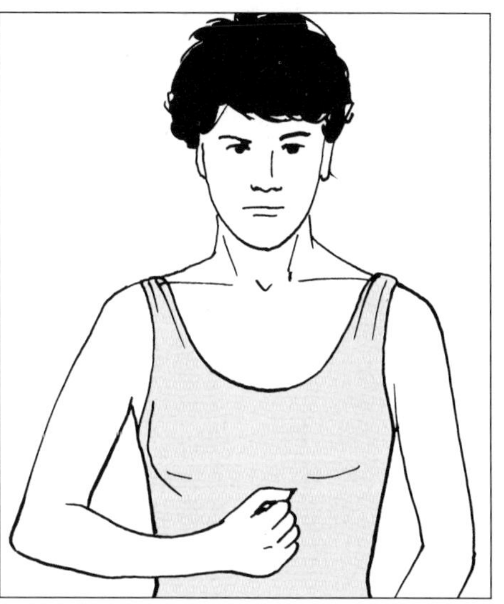

Mobility exercises

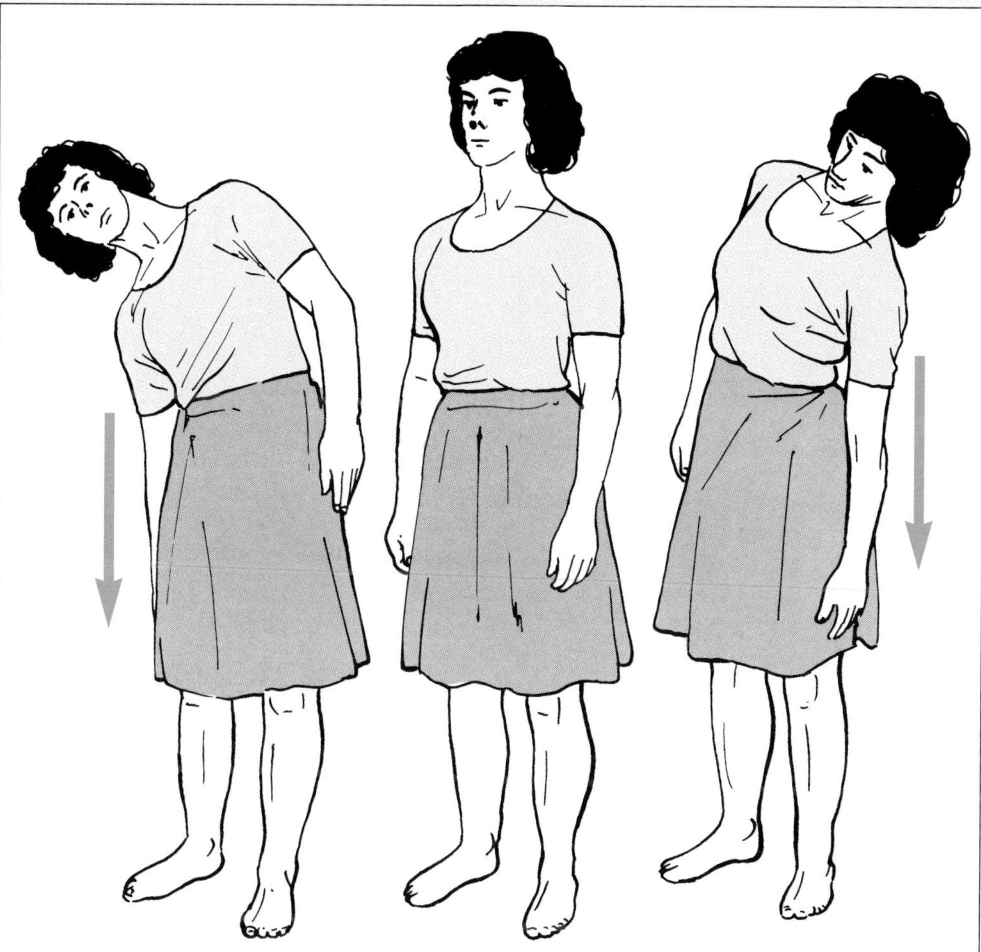

Stand with feet apart and your back against a wall, arms at sides. Slowly slide your right arm down your leg as far as feels comfortable. Slide back slowly to the original position and repeat on the other side. Repeat 5 times each side.

Mobility exercises

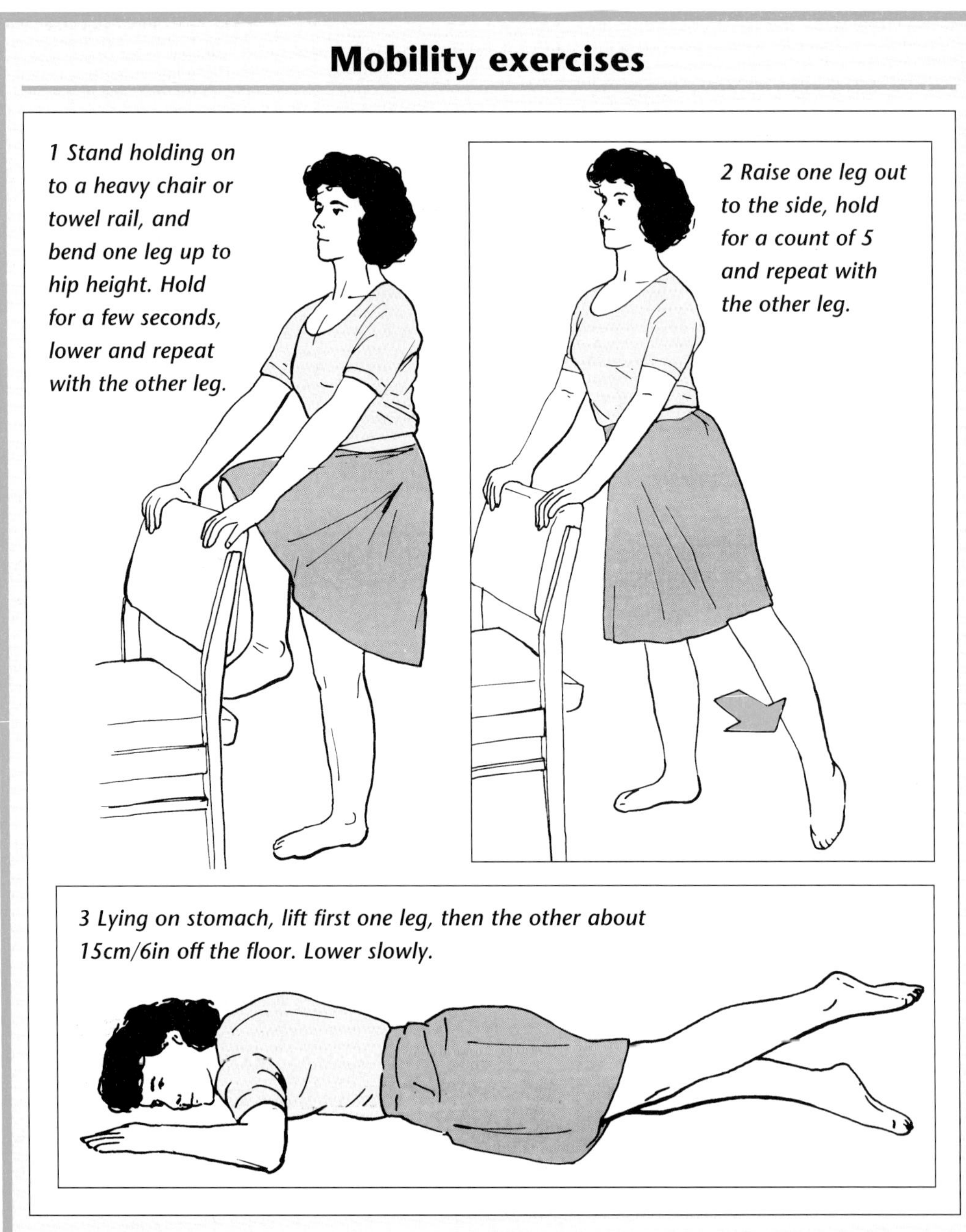

Mobility exercises

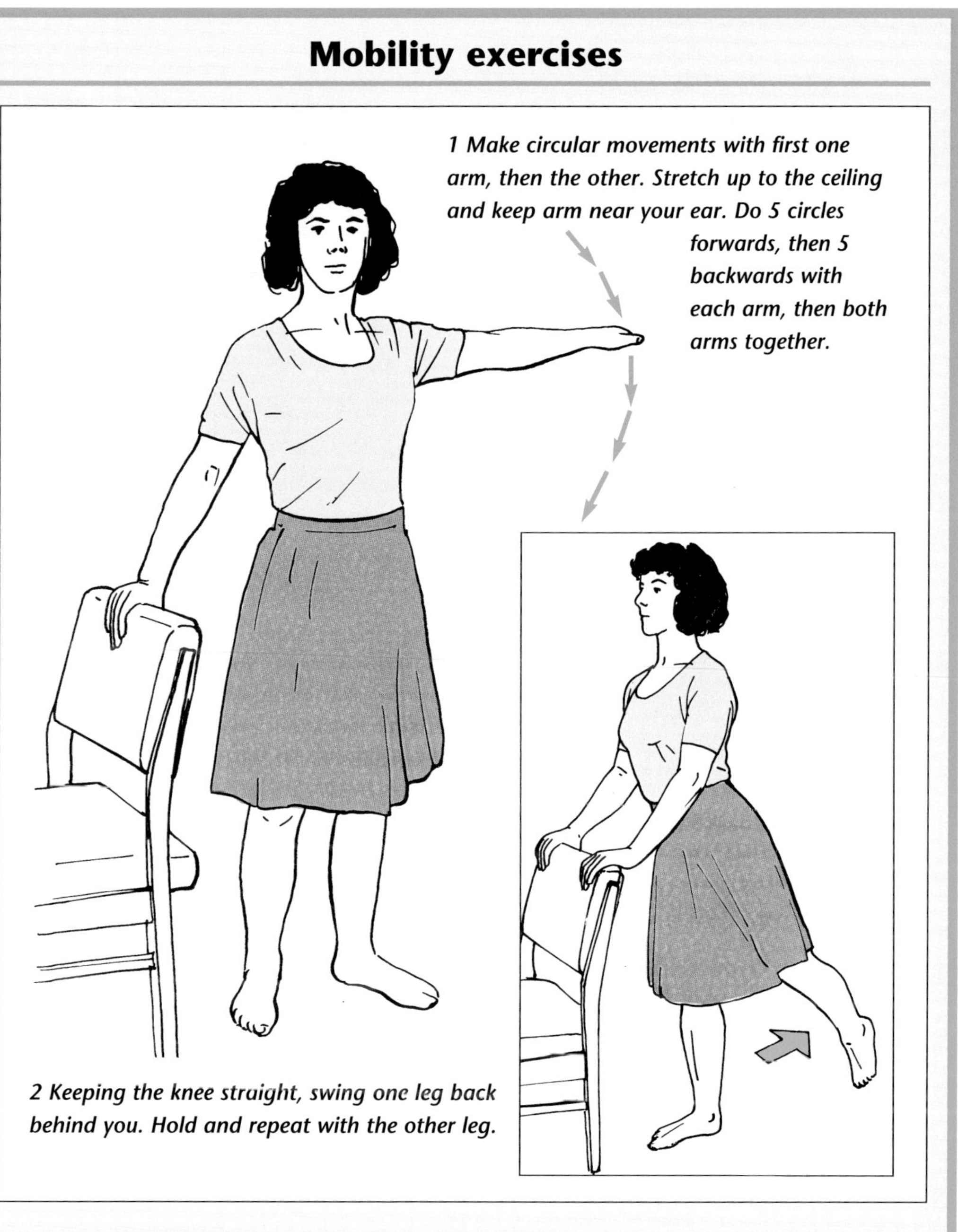

1 Make circular movements with first one arm, then the other. Stretch up to the ceiling and keep arm near your ear. Do 5 circles forwards, then 5 backwards with each arm, then both arms together.

2 Keeping the knee straight, swing one leg back behind you. Hold and repeat with the other leg.

Mobility exercises

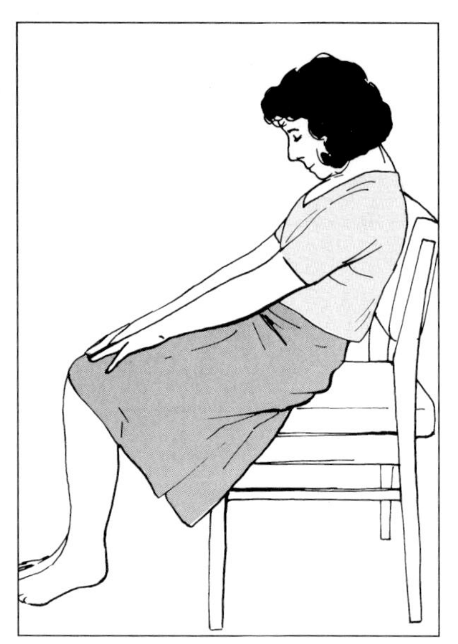

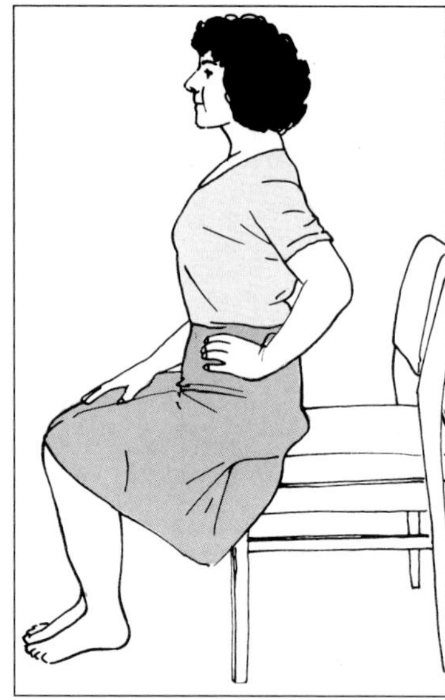

1 Sit up straight on a hard chair and allow the lower part of your spine to sag. Straighten your spine to create a small curve at the base.

2 With fingertips resting on shoulders, bring arms forwards and inwards until elbows touch. Move arms out and back as far as you can go, then circle them.

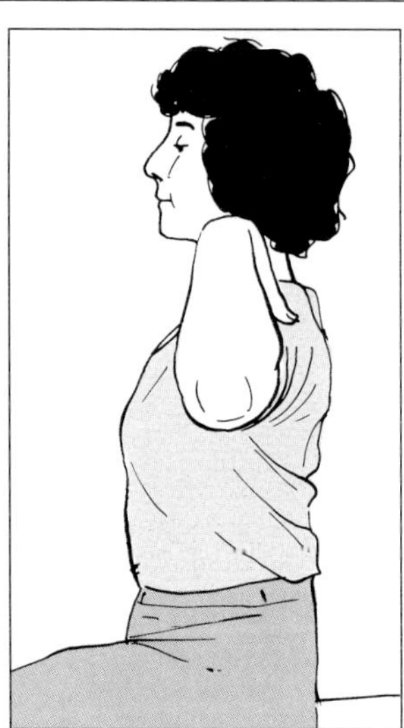

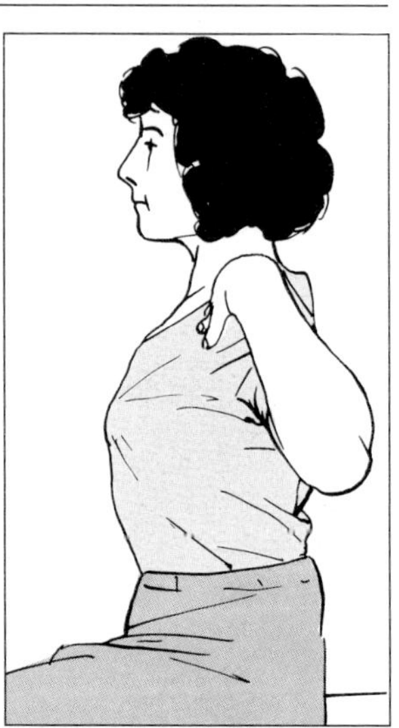

Mobility exercises

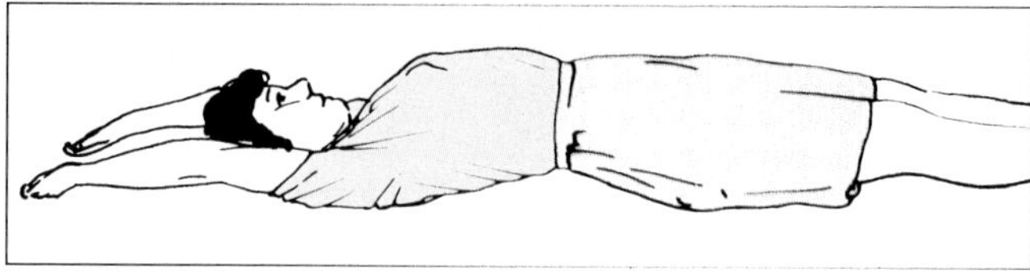

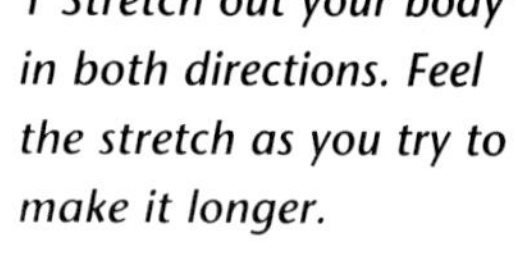

1 Stretch out your body in both directions. Feel the stretch as you try to make it longer.

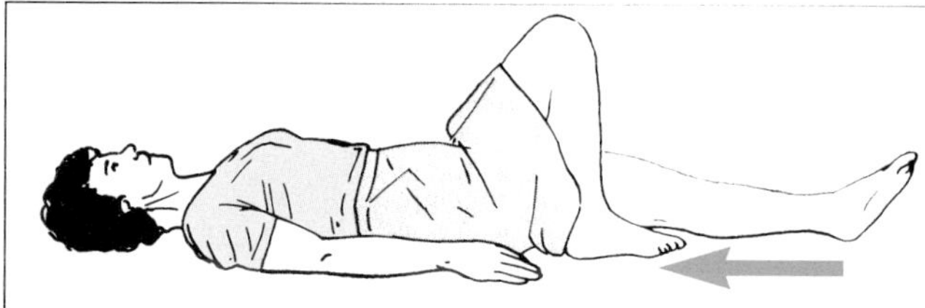

2 Hands at sides, slide one foot along the floor, bending your hip and knee towards you. Slowly lower and repeat on the other side.

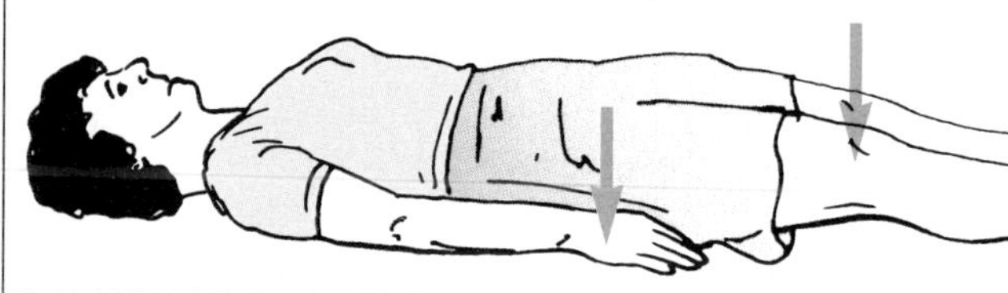

3 Push hands and knees down, simultaneously tightening your back, buttock and thigh muscles.

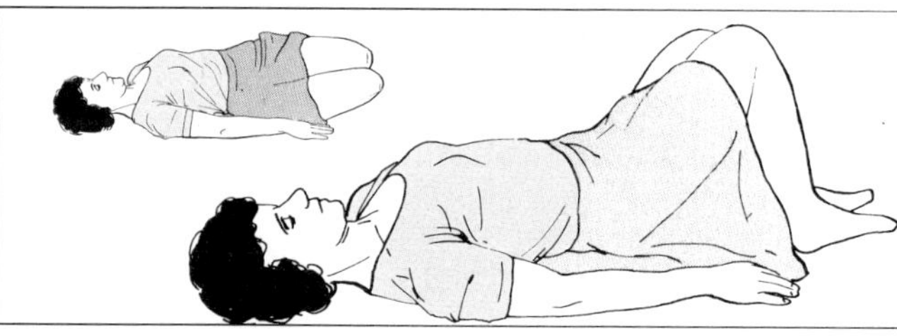

4 With arms at sides, roll your knees (keeping them together) to one side and then to the other. Move from the waist only – not the upper body.

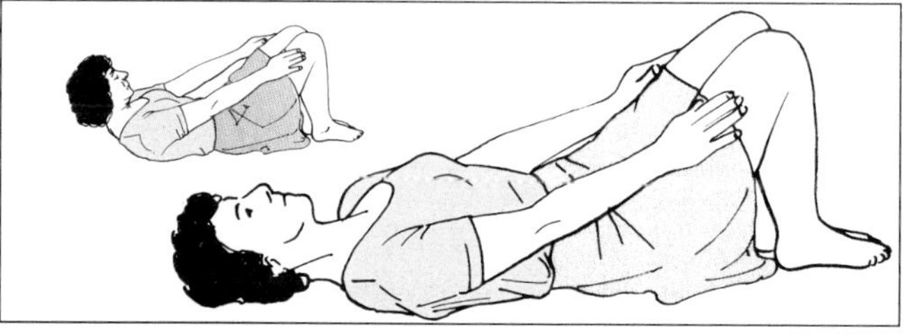

5 Lie on floor with knees bent and hands on thighs. Gradually lift head and shoulders off floor, sliding hands up towards knees. Gently lower head to the floor.

Chapter nine

Alternative therapies

There are many ways in which women can help themselves. The menopause is a perfectly natural phenomenon and one which responds to natural remedies. If you are uncertain about the vast range of alternative therapies around today, research to find out more about them will be worth the effort. It is important to stress here that, for more years than you care to admit, you have probably neglected your body. Women are often guilty of looking after everyone else except themselves. Now you need to take better care of you. It is no longer sensible to take your body for granted – not if you want to enjoy quality time. The next three decades have every chance of being the best years of your life but only if you slap a conservation order on yourself.

Hot flushes and night sweats

Some women find a vitamin E supplement, especially in combination with ginseng, gives a boost to the production of their natural oestrogen. Siberian rather than Korean ginseng is said to be better for hot flushes. Fennel oil is supposed to stimulate the production of oestrogen but you should only dabble with something as powerful as that in consultation with a skilled herbalist who, like homeopaths, treats the whole person. He or she will have experience of your particular symptoms and be able to advise about dosage, which is important because some herbs are particularly potent. If the flushes are accompanied by piercing headaches cranial osteopathy may help. Only go to a fully qualified practitioner. Other natural preparations to relieve these menopausal symptoms, available from some chemists and health food stores, include:

- Meltrosia.
- Belladonna.
- Pulsatilla.
- Sage.

Sex, loss of libido, feeling unloved

Some women swear by natural, live yogurt. Applied inside the vagina it can be soothing, can ward off infections and decrease dryness. Lubricants will help with initial penetration though prolonged intercourse may still be difficult as the beneficial effects rapidly disappear.

Fewer than 10 per cent of women suffer

from dyspareunia (pain related to sexual intercourse) and research has proved that the more sexually active women are, the less vaginal atrophy they suffer, raising the possibility that sexual activity protects the vagina. (Masturbation has a similarly protective effect.) This could be simply by stretching it or by stimulating hormone production, an interesting theory but one which is awaiting proof.

If you seem to have lost interest in making love, has it occurred to you to read a good book? Not instead of having sex, but to aid your libido. The right book can get you into the right frame of mind. Whatever turns you on, as they say.

It is also worth paying more attention to your bedtime routine. How do you look? Satin pyjamas or curlers and sticky face cream? Is the bedroom a boudoir or a tip? Indulge in some sexy sheets, scented candles or pretty lace pillows and curtains, not just for his benefit, but for yours, too.

Millions of women don't have a partner to have sex with so it is probably healthier for them to have a low or no libido. But feeling unloved is another matter altogether. Do you make people feel welcome? Do you go out of your way to make friends? Do you write that letter, make that phone call? There is nothing wrong with being a cantankerous old bat so long as you are not crabby all the time to everyone. Warm friendships are just as rewarding as hot affairs but they need nurturing.

Products to help

For practical products which will help you to overcome some of the mechanical trials and tribulations of making love if you are having difficulties during the menopause, look in a good chemist or health shop for:

- Senselle.
- KY Jelly.
- Sepia.
- Pulsatilla.
- Staphisagria.

OR try:

- Hypnosis.
- Yoga.
- Aromatherapy.

Insomnia, tiredness, exhaustion

These are among the most debilitating and self-perpetuating side-effects of growing older and the menopause. Almost any massage, particularly aromatherapy, will help. So will yoga and exercise, surprising though this may seem – and perhaps difficult to do if you are exhausted. But a brisk walk or gentle run before you go to bed will help you to sleep far more than watching television.

Never eat late at night: 7pm should be the latest and certainly don't drink tea or coffee. Try an infusion of passiflora (passion-fruit flowers). Have a warm bath and add three drops each of basil and cypress; three drops of thyme and rosemary; or three drops of rosemary, camomile and basil. Then, if you can bear it, have a cold shower. This stimulates the circulation and besides having an instant tingling effect is believed to have a beneficial long-term effect on the heart.

The following herbs or oils (many of them can be bought as scented candles or oil to put on asbestos rings and placed on top of light bulbs to scent the room) will also help to re-energise you:

- Meltrosia.
- Avena sativa, an extract of oats.
- Arnica.
- Camphor.
- Camomile.
- Jasmine.
- Marjoram.
- Neroli.
- Dr Bach's Flower Remedies.
- Curzon.
- Valerian.
- Dr Vogel's Dormeasan.

Mood swings, stress, irritability

These can be helped greatly by being kind to yourself. I know that sounds odd but women often neglect themselves thinking they are too busy to bother. But it sometimes makes them appear guilty of the martyr syndrome which does them no good at all and is not endearing. If you can afford it, have a massage, at least one every other month, if not more often. Or buy a book about massage: and teach yourself how to bring yourself relief by concentrating on certain critical pressure points. Shiatsu is like acupuncture without needles, which I thoroughly recommend. Other natural remedies you might like to try are:

- Biophylin.
- Newrelax.
- Aconitea.
- Lycopodium.
- Ignatia.
- Cimicifuga (Acte racemosa).
- Hepar Sulph.
- Sepia.
- Vitamin B6.
- Evening primrose oil .
- Dr Vogel's Formula MNP.

Finally

If you are still fed up about the menopause, and you haven't already done so, read Germaine Greer's book, *The Change*. It is funny, erudite and uncompromising. You will put it down whistling a happy tune.

Useful information

Marie Stopes Clinic
Marie Stopes Clinics were established in 1925 by the family planning pioneer. Today as an international charity, they provide a range of health services, including specialist Menopause Clinics. Clients are invited to have full check-ups with menopause experts, time to talk about the menopause symptoms, and advice and help on treatments, including all types of HRT. Fees are charged, and an information pack is available.

Marie Stopes Clinic (London)
108 Whitfield Street
London
W1P 6BE

Tel: London: 071 388 0662
Tel: Leeds: 0532 440685
Tel: Manchester: 061 832 4260

The Amarant Trust
80 Lambeth Road
London SE1 7PW
Tel: 071 401 3855

British Menopause Society
83 High Street
Marlow
Buckinghamshire SL7 1AB
Tel: 0761 32472

College of Homeopathy
26 Clarendon Rise
London SE13 5EY
Tel: 081 582 0573

Hormonal Health Care Centre
101 Harley Street
London W1

International Federation of Aromatherapists
Royal Masonic Hospital
Ravenscourt Park
London W6 0TN

Osteopathic Medical Association
22 Wimpole Street
London W1M 7AD
Tel: 071 323 4810

National Osteoporosis Society
PO Box 10
Radstock
Bath BA3 3YB
Tel: 0761 432472

Yoga Biomedical Trust
156 Cockerell Road
Cambridge

Index